D0877675

An Optometrist's Guide to Clinical Ethics

Edited by

R. Norman Bailey, OD

Elizabeth Heitman, PhD

American Optometric Association
St. Louis, Missouri

Library of Congress Card Number: 00-100874

ISBN 0-9700061-0-1

American Optometric Association
243 North Lindbergh Boulevard
St. Louis, MO 63141-7881

Honored to support the

advancement of clinical

ethics in optometry

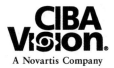

An Optometrist's Guide to Clinical Ethics was made possible by a grant from CIBA Vision—A Novartis Company

Contents

- False-positive and false-negative results
- The benefits and harms of diagnostic information
- Confidentiality, discrimination, and conflict of interest
  References

**7 Allocation of Resources and Relations with   61
Third-Party Payers**
Michael Larkin, OD

- Technology, staffing, and the optometrist's role in patient care
- Medical necessity and quality of care
- Managed care and capitation
- Utilization review and denial of coverage
- Auditing and other contract issues
  References

8 Adopting New Equipment, Techniques, and Technology 73
Arthur H. Alexander, OD

- Acquiring new equipment and devices
- The cost of new devices
- Introduction of new technology into practice
- The genomics revolution
  References

**Part II   SPECIAL POPULATIONS AND SPECIAL
ETHICAL PROBLEMS IN OPTOMETRIC PRACTICE**

9 Children and Adolescents   87
Dawn C. Kaufman, OD & LeRoy Kaufman, OD

- Consent, assent, and refusal of treatment
- Privacy and confidentiality

Preface

This text is intended to serve both as a broad discussion of the ethical issues inherent in the clinical practice of optometry and as a general reference for optometrists who seek guidance in dealing with ethical questions and conflicts in patient care. It is not meant to give "the answer" to the question of what actions to take in given ethical situations arising in clinical practice. Rather, it offers insights and a decision-making process that can guide the practitioner toward an appropriate course of action when facing an ethical issue in practice. The original motivation for this book came from the Ethics Education Program for Optometric Practitioners, which identified the need for a comprehensive text on the ethical issues of clinical optometry. Ethical concerns related to the business aspects of optometric practice, while important, are not within the intended scope of this text.

The material in this book was commissioned and reviewed by the American Optometric Association Ethics and Values Committee, which supports the consideration of diverse perspectives on ethical issues in clinical practice. Individuals with professional backgrounds in optometry and ethics, from both academics and private practice, have written the essays included here. Although the American Optometric Association (AOA) has sponsored this project, the individual essays reflect the opinions of their respective authors and others consulted in their preparation, and do not necessarily represent the views of the AOA.

While we have constructed this text to be an off-the-shelf reference for practicing ODs, we hope that it will also be a useful tool in the professional education of future optometrists studying in the schools and colleges of optometry. The cases presented as examples of ethical issues in clinical practice are suitable for analysis and discussion by optometric practitioners and optometry students at all levels. These cases are fictional and were written specifically for inclusion in this volume. Any similarity between the circumstances or characters described in these cases and actual events involving actual persons, living or dead, is purely coincidental.

We are aware that projects and programs of the AOA often impact the practice of optometry worldwide. This influence is both an honor and a

great responsibility. Although this book addresses the practice of optometry in the United States, we hope that it will encourage optometrists in
other countries to consider questions of professional behavior in their own
national contexts and promote high ethical standards for the profession
worldwide.

We are extremely grateful to have had the opportunity to work with the
many people who have been involved in this project as it moved through
its various stages. We regret that we were unable to call upon the many
other individuals who also would have been capable of making significant
contributions to this work. We encourage everyone who reads these essays
to become actively involved in the promotion of professional values and
behavior among their peers. Optometry needs its members to speak out on
ethical issues in a collegial and supportive way to guide the profession
through its second century. Contemplation of the professional values and
obligations addressed in this book should strengthen optometrists' collective resolve to maintain the highest ethical standards for the benefit of all
patients.

We hope that you enjoy reading this book as much as the editors and
members of the Ethics and Values Committee enjoyed taking part in its
development. Because both the fields of optometry and ethics continue to
develop, no book on optometric ethics can be definitive. If you believe that
specific topics should be added or expanded to enhance the value of the
text, please forward your suggestions to the editors in care of the AOA. All
such comments will be considered for possible future revisions.

R. Norman Bailey, OD
Elizabeth Heitman, PhD
Houston, Texas
October 1999

Acknowledgments

It is with great pleasure that I take this opportunity to recognize those who have played a major role in bringing this significant project of the Ethics and Values Committee of the American Optometric Association (AOA) to its full realization. Several years ago, the Ethics and Values Committee began to contemplate various projects that could support the Ethics Education Program for Optometric Practitioners. The need to create a text to encourage continued high ethical standards in optometric clinical practice seemed to be foremost in the Committee's discussion.

A nationally recognized health care ethicist was engaged to assist the Committee in planning the content of such a text, as well as the process of bringing together a group of expert optometrists as authors. From the beginning, the Committee sought to develop a book that could be of significant value to the members of the AOA and to the students of the schools and colleges of optometry. Over the past few years the members of the Committee have played the major role of developing the project concept, commissioning the editors and authors, and reviewing the chapter manuscripts. From the initial project discussions to publication of the text, the following Committee members are recognized for their various contributions over the past several years: Drs. Robert P. Aitken, Arthur H. Alexander, Nancy Barr, Donovan L. Crouch, Thomas F. Dorrity, Jr., Alden N. Haffner, Rick T. Iwai, Linda Johnson, Robert W. McCullough, James E. Paramore, Alessi A. Rispoli, and Laurie L. Sorrenson.

The optometrist authors of the individual chapters deserve both recognition and praise for their insights into the many professional obligations and ethical issues impacting optometric practice, as well for as their generous donation of time and energy to the book project. All have contributed without financial remuneration, and are to be thanked for their wonderful gift to the readers of this text and to the profession as a whole. They include: Drs. Arthur H. Alexander, Thomas F. Dorrity, Jr., Kia B. Eldred, N. Scott Gorman, Elizabeth Hoppe, Dawn C. Kaufman, LeRoy Kaufman, Brian S. Klinger, Michael Larkin, Edwin C. Marshall, Mark Swanson, Satya B. Verma, and Siu G. Wong.

The essential contributions of our ethicist consultants, Drs. Elizabeth Heitman and David T. Ozar, have added considerable credibility to the work. Dr. Heitman's specific contributions will be recognized later. Dr. Ozar served as both an author and a general consultant on issues of professionalism and professional ethics. Over the past several years, the Chair and Staff of the Ethics and Values Committee have consulted him on several occasions. He has also served as a consultant to the Optometric Ethics Educators Special Interest Group of the Association of Schools and Colleges of Optometry.

The AOA staff contributed both time and expertise toward many aspects of the project, and their efforts were essential to the success of the final volume. In particular, grateful acknowledgment is due to Leon Carslick, Administrative Assistant in the Office of Counsel; Sherry Cooper, Legal Research Associate; Judith DuChateau, JD, AOA Associate Counsel; Thomas E. Eichhorst, JD, AOA Counsel, and the staff of the AOA Communications Group who were instrumental in the publication and distribution of the text, especially Andrew L. Miller, Associate Director — Publications and Kimberly Stuckmeyer, Production Designer. Thanks are also due to other staff in the St. Louis and Washington, DC offices and the staff of the International Library, Archives and Museum of Optometry (ILAMO) for their fact checking and contributions to the accuracy of references.

Simple words of acknowledgment and appreciation seem inadequate when recognizing the contribution that our primary ethics consultant and my co-editor, Elizabeth Heitman, made to this project. Her expertise and professional experience in health care ethics and editing are evident throughout the text. She helped a diverse group of optometric practitioners express their ideas in a way that gives continuity to the final volume. Through her work with this and other Ethics and Values Committee projects during the past several years, she has learned much about the clinical practice of optometry and the ethical values that are the underpinning of our daily professional activities. In turn, she has helped me and many others explore and articulate the ethical ideals of optometry in ways that enrich the profession as a whole.

Kevin L. Alexander, OD, PhD, AOA Board Liaison Trustee to the Ethics and Values Committee of the Clinical Care Group, is gratefully thanked for his review of the final manuscript.

Finally, CIBA Vision Corporation – a Novartis Company, has played an essential role as financial sponsor of this project, enabling it to move forward from its early planning stages. Their generous grant has provided the necessary funds to develop, publish, print, and distribute this text free of charge to all optometrist members of the AOA and to all third and fourth year optometry students in North America. CIBA Vision Corporation, and particularly Richard E. Weisbarth, OD, CIBA's Executive Director of Professional Services for North America, has been a supporter of high ethical standards in the optometric profession for many years. In 1995 CIBA, through Dr. Weisbarth's foresight, provided a grant to the AOA Ethics and Values Committee that enabled the AOA to assist the Optometric Ethics Educators, chaired by Dr. Leonard Werner of the State College of Optometry of the State University of New York, in the development of the Recommended Curriculum for the Teaching of Professionalism and Ethics in Optometry for use in the schools and colleges of optometry. We are most appreciative of CIBA Vision Corporation's ongoing assistance, and gratefully acknowledge their important role in advancing the values of the optometric profession.

R. Norman Bailey, OD, Chair
Ethics and Values Committee
American Optometric Association

Message from the President

In my presidential inaugural address in San Antonio in June 1999, I noted: "It is the AOA's job to enhance and promote the independent and ethical decision making of its members and to assist doctors of optometry in practicing successfully in accordance with the highest standards of patient care."

This book is yet another example of the informational materials and services that the AOA provides to its member optometrists and optometry students in the fulfillment of that pledge of assistance.

After contemplating the circumstances presented in the case studies and then studying the narrative of the chapters of this book, we as professional optometrists will be better prepared to discern and properly consider ethical issues that present themselves in clinical practice.

The profession of optometry, and the patients we all serve, will benefit greatly from the increased attention to the ethical concepts this book will invite and direct. My congratulations to the O.D. authors, and especially to the optometric editor, Dr. Norman Bailey, all of whom donated their services in this noble endeavor.

I am also appreciative of the continuing support of CIBA Vision Corporation—a Novartis Company, which has provided the funding for the production and dissemination of this work.

As the 1999–2000 President of the American Optometric Association, I am pleased and proud to present to the profession *An Optometrist's Guide to Clinical Ethics*. This valuable addition to the literature of our profession will be of great help to each of us as we individually strive to always achieve the first precept of the AOA Code of Ethics—"To keep the visual welfare of the patient uppermost at all times."

Harvey P. Hanlen, OD
President
American Optometric Association

Professional Obligations and Optometry

David T. Ozar, PhD

Questions about how we ought to act arise in every aspect of human life. This book has been written specifically to assist its readers in their professional lives. Optometry is one of the *professions* and optometrists view themselves and are viewed by their patients as *professionals*. The ideas of *profession* and *professional* add important considerations to the theme of ethical decision making.

To begin, it is useful to identify some of the characteristics of professions and professionals that make optometry a profession and an individual optometrist a professional. Among the most important characteristics of professions and professionals are these four:

First, each profession possesses a distinctive expertise that consists of both theoretical knowledge and the skills necessary to apply that knowledge in practice. To be accepted as a member of a profession, an individual must master the profession's expertise to a sufficient degree that he or she can be depended on to routinely apply it correctly without direct supervision.

Second, this combination of theoretical knowledge and the skills for applying it is a necessary means to the achievement of some class of important benefits for members of the larger community, in their individual lives or collectively.

Third, the acquisition of such expertise ordinarily depends upon extensive theoretical study and training under the direction of persons already a part of the profession. The expertise of a profession is typically exclusive to the members of the profession. Those who are not members are typically unable to make timely and dependable judgments in matters pertaining to the profession's expertise.

And fourth, because members of a profession are recognized by the larger community as possessing expertise and because such expertise is ordinarily exclusive to the members, judgments pertaining to the profession's expertise are usually made by its members. This fact grants a great amount of autonomy to the professions, as decisions made by their members are ordinarily accepted as authoritative within the larger community.

Nonetheless, a community does not automatically accept the authority of an individual's or group's judgments about something simply because the person or group had undergone intensive training or is considered expert. Instead, a community might actually be very cautious if it fears that the expert group might use its exclusive expertise solely for the benefit of its members, or even hold the community hostage to their expertise. This risk would be the greatest when, as in the case of most professions, those outside the expert group simply do not have enough understanding of what is at stake to make dependable judgments about it, or to do so quickly enough to take appropriate action.

So it is worth asking under what circumstances a society would be acting reasonably to routinely accept the judgments of persons with important, specialized expertise as authoritative. What would justify such a measure of trust of an expert group whose judgments cannot practically be tested because they depend on expertise that others do not have? What sort of social structure could effectively safeguard a community from the potential harms of an expert group's misuse of its expertise?

The answer to this question in the case of the professions is the complex social structure that we call *professional obligation* or, when it is a characteristic of a profession or an individual professional, *professionalism*. That is to say, there is a fifth core characteristic of professions and professionals that is, for present purposes, the most important:

Professions and professionals have special obligations precisely because they are professionals. Becoming a member of a profession implies acceptance of a set of standards of professional conduct by that person, both in personal commitment and in actual practice.

Some people take the view that practicing a profession is no different in principle from selling one's wares in the marketplace. According to this view, a professional has a product to sell and makes agreements with interested purchasers, and that is all there is to it. Beyond some fundamental obligation not to coerce, cheat, or defraud others, which are the ethics of the marketplace, this view holds that a professional has no other obligations to anyone except those undertaken in voluntary agreements with specific individuals or groups. According to this picture, in other words, there is nothing to which a person is obligated precisely because he or she is a professional.

But most people in our society and most professionals themselves hold that when a group becomes a profession, or when an individual becomes a member of a profession, they undertake obligations to act and refrain from acting in certain ways. Otherwise, the community and its members would have no good reason to trust the profession and its members to use their exclusive expertise appropriately. Fortunately, our society has extensive positive experience with professional obligation and professionalism. The social structure of the professions has effectively shaped the behavior of professionals so that appropriate conduct is typical and aberrations are relatively rare. Thus the relationship of trust upon which the mutual flourishing of both the professions and the larger community genuinely depends has been maintained.

Each profession has expertise that addresses specific aspects of human well-being, either individual or collective; and each profession has distinctive relationships with those whom it serves. In one sense, the content of a professional's ethical life – what aspects of life the professional takes to be ethically important, and the standards of conduct by which the professional determines how to act, especially when actually engaged in professional practice – is distinctive for each profession. Optometry has its own ethical standards; it is not medicine, nor law, nor dentistry, engineering, journalism, or any other profession.

But there are common patterns across the professions from which each of the professions can learn. There are core questions that can be asked of every profession that will enable its members to articulate more clearly the content of their profession's ethical standards and, therefore, their professional obligations.

What describes the ethical norms for optometry? Optometrists' ethical norms are described in the American Optometric Association Code of Ethics and Standards of Conduct, and the Optometric Oath. These documents are an important starting point for examining the ethics of the optometric profession. They are expressions of the content of optometry's ethics that have been discussed and approved by many thoughtful optometrists over the years. But the content of every profession's ethics is much richer and subtler than the text of a published code or other sets of standards can articulate, just as the organizations that publish such documents are never fully representative of all of a given profession's practitioners. It is, therefore, very important for the members of a profession to examine such published statements periodically to see when anything important has been left out or if the changing circumstances of the profession's practice over time have made new ethical issues important enough that they should be covered in published codes or standards.

The experienced practitioner of any profession typically understands far more about the ethical practice of his or her profession than a published code or set of standards could ever say. Unfortunately, as in many professions, members of the optometric profession have not often carefully articulated their understanding of the role of professional ethics in specific areas of their practice. This book aims to move this process forward by inviting thoughtful practitioners to do just that. Each reader of this book should do this personally as well, not only reading and reflecting on the essays, but also formulating his or her answers to the questions that every profession's ethic implicitly tries to answer.

Sources of Professional Obligations

The various professions all try to respond in their ethical systems to a set of core questions.[1] The effort to answer these questions carefully for optometry will be a most valuable self-education exercise for the optometrist who reads this book. Here are nine core questions:

Who are this profession's *chief clients*?

The *chief client* is the set of persons whose well-being the profession and its members are chiefly committed to serving. Whose well-being are optometry and the individual optometrist chiefly committed to serving?

There is no convenient word in English to use to refer in general terms to the beneficiary of professional services. "Beneficiary" is a very clumsy word; "client" may suggest to some a merely commercial, rather than a professional, relationship. Since optometry is a health profession, there is an appropriate word to use for this purpose, namely, "patient."

But who are the patients that optometry is committed to serving? Only the patient in the chair? Surely not, because there are patients in the reception room to whom the optometrist has professional obligations as well. Then there are all of the optometrist's patients of record. There are emergency patients. And there is the whole community, toward whom the optometrist has obligations in several respects. Answering this question will take some careful thinking; and the same is true of the other questions as well. But if these questions *are* answered carefully, the result will reveal ethical features of almost every aspect of daily optometric practice.

What is the *ideal relationship* between a member of the profession and the client?

The purpose of the relationship between a professional and a client is to bring about certain values for the client. Bringing about these values requires both the professional and the client to make judgments and choices about the professional's interventions. What are the proper roles of the professional and the client, particularly in regard to these judgments and choices?

The short, too-easy answer to this question for optometry is that the relationship between the optometrist and the patient must be one of informed consent. But is this truly the *ideal relationship* that optometrists should always aim for or is it, rather, the bare minimum below which they ought not fall? Could the *ideal relationship* be one of close collaboration between patient and professional in the judgments and choices involved in treatment? In either case, what is the proper relationship when something less than the ideal is all that is possible, as when the patient is a child, is developmentally disabled, or is otherwise not fully capable of participating as a decision maker? Most practitioners take these matters very seriously. But articulating what they do in practice, what the ethical optometrist aims at in relating to a patient, and what sorts of interpersonal skills are needed to do so, involves far more than naming the minimal legal standard of informed consent.

What are the *central values* of this profession?

No profession can realistically be committed to securing for its clients everything that is of value for them. Rather, there is a certain set of values that are the focus of each profession's special expertise and which it is, therefore, the job and obligation of that profession to work to secure for its clients. These are the professions' *central or core values*.

The short, too-easy answer to this question for optometry is the health of the eye and good vision for the patient. But both *health* and *good vision* are concepts for which there are not simple, obvious meanings already available to optometry. Nor can either of these crucial concepts be simply scientifically defined. What characteristics of vision are judged *good*, or otherwise, for a given individual depends on what is physically possible for that individual and on what is needed, expected, demanded of that individual within his or her environment. Both of these factors are in turn affected by larger social values and expectations. The same is true, although often in even more subtle ways, of concepts of *health*.

In addition, the optometrist must ask whether he or she would be practicing in a professionally ethical manner if ocular health and good vision were the *only* values that he or she attended to. Optometrists have obligations regarding the patient's *general health* and even the patient's *life* insofar as, for example, the eye and its surrounding structures can manifest relevant patterns of signs and symptoms that have broader ramifications. Optometrists arguably have obligations to attend to patients' *autonomy* insofar as this important value is at stake in various aspects of their mutual decision making. One might also ask whether optometrists have obligations to patients regarding the *esthetics* of their appearance, or whether the esthetic aspects of vision correction are merely optional matters in professional optometric practice. There is again much in good ethical optometric practice that could be better articulated.

What are the norms of *competence* of this profession?

Every profession is obligated both to acquire and to maintain the expertise needed to benefit clients in the tasks that it routinely undertakes, and in which it represents itself to be expert. Every professional similarly must acquire and maintain the expertise that characterizes the profession. Individual professionals are obligated to undertake only those tasks that are within their own competence, and to assist clients whose needs lie outside that competence by locating another professional who can assist them.

The practical skill of knowing when a patient's specific presenting condition is beyond one's competence, the habit of routinely watching for such circumstances, and the courage and honesty needed to act appropriately when such circumstances arise are character traits of considerable subtlety. How should the ethical optometrist recognize the limits of his or her competence, and how should he or she appropriately convey to patients that they must seek another's assistance?

Related to this matter is the larger issue of maintaining the competence of the profession as a whole. How carefully does the profession monitor its individual practitioners and how does it respond when something has gone wrong? What should individual optometrists do when they observe possible incompetent practice by another optometrist? What standards of evidence and degree of possible harm to patients should determine how they react? Each of the health professions also has a profound responsibility to influence the views of the larger community about what constitutes good health and ill health and what counts as competent intervention in relation to health care.

How much *sacrifice* is required of the members of this profession and in what aspects of their professional lives? How much *priority* – and under what circumstances – does the well-being of the profession's clients have over other morally relevant considerations affecting its members?

Professions are regularly characterized as being committed to the service and best interest of their clients and the general public. But these expressions permit many different interpretations with very different implications for actual practice. It is important to ask just what measure of sacrifice of personal interest and of the professional's other commitments is professionally obligatory.

Every profession's ethics involves sacrifices on the part of its members for the sake of those whom the profession serves. An optometrist who claimed he or she had no such obligations would be in error. But at the same time, even though many health professions' published documents claim that the patient's well-being is *always the highest priority*, it is unreasonable to think that this is literally true. It is unreasonable to think that the professional's obligation to sacrifice other values, including commitments to other persons, are always absolutely overridden by the patient's well-being or the profession's *central values*. Careful reflection is needed to identify more clearly what sorts of sacrifices optometrists are and are not professionally called upon to make for the sake of their patients.

What is the *ideal relationship* between the members of this profession and *co-professionals*?

Each profession also has norms, typically implicit and unexamined, concerning the proper relationship between members of the same profession in various matters as well as between members of different professions who deal with the same clients. Included under this heading for optometry, for example, are questions about the proper relationships between optometrists and ophthalmologists, other physicians, and other health professionals caring for the same patients, as well the relationships among optometrists themselves on many matters that affect patient care and patients' access to care in various ways. Here, too, arise questions about ethically proper ways of interacting with employees who assist the optometrist in the care of patients and who therefore are representatives to patients of the optometrist's ethical commitments.

What is the *ideal relationship* between the members of this profession and *the larger community*?

Besides relationships between professionals and their clients and professionals with one another, the activities of every profession also involve relationships between the profession as a group and the larger community as a whole or its various significant subgroups. Here the obligations of professional organizations need to be considered, including questions of whom such organizations are supposed to serve and the values that are supposed to underlie this service. Individual professionals likely have relationships with individual members or groups within the larger community who are neither co-professionals nor patients. These relationships come in many forms and may be focused on issues unrelated to professional practice. A professional is obligated to examine these relationships regularly to determine whether and how they affect his or her obligations to patients or the obligations of the profession as a whole. Each optometric professional also has an obligation to the larger community to help maintain and improve both the competence of the profession of optometry as a whole and the extent to which it lives by appropriate ethical standards. Meeting these obligations most often means working within the profession, but may sometimes mean working outside of it as well.

What are the profession and its members obligated to do to *secure access* to the benefits of their expertise for all those in need within their society?

Although implicitly addressed elsewhere, the ethical issue of justly distributing the profession's services to those who need them deserves explicit attention in the articulation of the profession's ethic. Most members of the optometric profession provide some measure of uncompensated care to patients who would not receive appropriate eye and vision care otherwise. But there may be other actions that an optometrist concerned with patients' lack of access to appropriate visual health care might appropriately take in our society. Determining what sorts of action might be professionally required, both for individual patients and in regard to political or social action, is an ethically serious issue for every practitioner. Undertaking appropriate social and political action should also be part of the agenda of professional organizations as they examine their ethical obligations.

What are the members of this profession obligated to do to preserve the *integrity* of their commitment to its values and to educate others about them?

Professional *integrity* includes the conduct by which a person communicates to others what he or she stands for, not only in acts themselves, but also in how these acts are chosen and in how the person presents himself or herself to others in carrying them out. It is a very important issue, for example, to ask whether a health professional has a special obligation to live in a healthy way, with the rationale that failing to do so models to the larger community a commitment to values inconsistent with life as a health professional. What aspects of an optometrist's life could members of the public, and especially the optometrist's patients, rightly look to as representing the values that the profession and its members stand for?

These nine questions, taken together, outline the central elements of the ethics of a profession. Reflecting on how to answer these questions for optometry and on scenarios in which the answers are played out can be a valuable and professionally enriching exercise. Discussing one's answers, and scenarios that exemplify them, with other members of the profession will spread the effort and improve not only the profession's practice of its ethics, but its unity and commitment to ethical practice as well. This volume of essays and cases offers the opportunity for just such professional discussion and reflection, and should be actively engaged by all its readers.

Reference

1. Ozar DT, Sokol DJ. *Dental ethics at the chairside: professional principles and practical applications.* Washington, DC: Georgetown University Press; copyright, Mosby-Yearbook, Inc., 1994.

Part I

GENERAL ETHICAL CONSIDERATIONS IN OPTOMETRIC PRACTICE

Chapter One

Ethics in Clinical Optometry

R. Norman Bailey, OD
Elizabeth Heitman, PhD

Health care professionals have long understood the fundamental responsibility that practitioners have toward their patients: in clinical practice, the well-being of the patient takes priority over all other issues. In this guide to clinical ethics, a variety of experienced optometrists and ethicists examine aspects of clinical optometry in which ethical questions may arise in the care of patients. Our purpose in this anthology is to introduce clinicians to ethical discourse on a variety of important topics in everyday practice in optometry, and to provide general guidance for optometrists faced with ethical questions in their own work. We hope to provide students of optometry as well as seasoned vision care specialists a systematic consideration of the ethics of clinical optometry based on the highest professional standards.

Reflection on ethical issues is an essential complement to professionals' specialized knowledge and skills in meeting basic human needs. Because professionals' knowledge and skills cannot be fully understood by those whom they serve, professions depend on the public's trust. To protect the public from practitioners who would take advantage of the vulnerable, and to safeguard the trust upon which professional practice is based, professional groups and associations have historically developed formal standards of behavior to guide the ethical conduct of their members. In health care these standards are often written as codes of ethics, which typically describe the ethical relationship that should exist between the caregiver and society, the doctor and professional colleagues and, most importantly, the doctor and patients.

Babylonian physicians had a written code of ethical principles and outlined the conduct required of the doctor nearly 4,500 years ago.[1] The

Hippocratic Oath,[2] attributed to the ancient Greek physician Hippocrates, continues to influence the behavior of health care practitioners today. The Hippocratic Oath laid out a number of essential values that have stood the test of time, including the primacy of the patient's welfare, the duty to avoid causing harm, and the preservation of confidentiality.[3,4]

Optometry has engaged in professional consideration of its ethical standards throughout its history, and the American Optometric Association (AOA) has worked to encourage professional behavior among practicing optometrists since its inception.[5] The AOA House of Delegates adopted its current Code of Ethics[6] at the 1944 Annual Congress. Other documents directing the ethical behavior of AOA members have been written and modified since that time. Currently, the AOA Code is supplemented by the Standards of Conduct[7] and the Optometric Oath,[8] which support and expand the ideas set forth in the Code.

The ethical obligations of optometry toward patients are similar to those of other health care professions.[9] These obligations generally require optometrists to recognize, respect, and protect the rights of their patients. This approach encourages patients to participate actively in their care and allows them to develop a relationship with their optometrist based on trust.

While the ethical principles under which the optometric profession functions have remained relatively constant, dramatic changes in technology, the scope of optometric practice, and the environment of health care delivery have created pressing new ethical questions in the clinical setting. Ethical conflicts are evident, for example, in the growing ability to diagnose conditions for which effective treatment is not available, in certain restrictions on treatment demanded by third-party insurers and managed care systems, and in the high costs of some emerging technologies.

Many ethical issues are affected by legal standards, and it is vital for optometrists to know the law relevant to their practice. But while the law provides an important set of guidelines for professional behavior, it is not always enough in specific situations. Due to the changing nature of practice, there may be significant lag between the first appearance of an ethical problem and the creation of appropriate legislation or case law to address it. Moreover, legislation may be too broad and case law too narrow to answer some practice questions clearly. Laws may also vary considerably from state to state. Finally, a practice that focuses too closely on avoiding the threat of malpractice litigation may view patients as adversaries rather than people in need. In the end, professionals are expected to be persons of integrity and judgment who go beyond the minimalist standards of the law in order to build and sustain trusting, therapeutic relationships.[10]

We hope that the essays in this collection will broaden the conversation on ethics in optometry to include a wide range of clinical topics. We encourage you to review the AOA Code of Ethics and Standards of Conduct, and The Optometric Oath below and, as you read the chapters that follow, consider your own practice and how these documents reflect the ethical standards of everyday clinical optometry.

Code of Ethics

It Shall Be the Ideal, the Resolve and the Duty of the Members of The American Optometric Association:

- TO KEEP the visual welfare of the patient uppermost at all times;

- TO PROMOTE in every possible way, in collaboration with this Association, better care of the visual needs of mankind;

- TO ENHANCE continuously their educational and technical proficiency to the end that their patients shall receive the benefits of all acknowledged improvements in visual care;

- TO SEE THAT no person shall lack for visual care, regardless of his financial status;

- TO ADVISE the patient whenever consultation with an optometric colleague or reference for other professional care seems advisable;

- TO HOLD in professional confidence all information concerning a patient and to use such data only for the benefit of the patient;

- TO CONDUCT themselves as exemplary citizens;

- TO MAINTAIN their offices and their practices in keeping with professional standards;

- TO PROMOTE and maintain cordial and unselfish relationships with members of their own profession and of other professions for the exchange of information to the advantage of mankind.

Standards of Conduct

I. Basic Responsibilities of An Optometrist

Section A. The Welfare of Humanity

A health profession has as its prime objective the service it can render to humanity; monetary considerations should be a subordinate factor. In choosing the profession of optometry an individual assumes an obligation for personal conduct in accordance with professional ideals.

Section B. Continuing Competence

An optometrist should strive to keep current with every modern development in the profession, to enhance both knowledge and proficiency by the adoption of modern methods and scientific concepts of proven worth and to contribute personally to the general knowledge and advancement of the profession. All these things should be done with that freedom of action and thought that provides first for the welfare of the public.

II. Relationship With The Patient

Section A. Informed Consent

An optometrist should provide to the patient sufficient information in order to obtain an informed consent from the patient.

Section B. Emergency Optometric Care

A request for optometric care in an emergency should receive immediate response. Once having undertaken an emergency case, an optometrist shall neither abandon nor neglect the patient.

Section C. Charges For Materials

Charges for materials should be clearly separated from professional fees.

III. Responsibilities To The Public

Section A. Informing The Public

An optometrist should honor the applicable provisions of valid State and Federal laws and rules regulating the advertising of ophthalmic materials and the disseminating of information regarding professional services.

IV. Relationships With Other Optometrists

Section A. Intraprofessional Referral And Consultations

Intraprofessional referral and consultations are encouraged when the best interest of the patient indicates additional opinion. Protocol on the relationship and responsibilities between the referring and attending optometrist that customarily is followed by health professions shall prevail.

Section B. Official Position

An optometrist holding an official position in any optometric organization shall avoid any semblance of using this position for self-aggrandizement.

V. Relationships With Other Professionals

Section A. Interprofessional Referral And Consultations

Interprofessional referral and consultations are encouraged when the best interest of the patient indicates additional opinion. Protocol on the relationship and responsibilities between the referring and attending professional that customarily is followed by health professions shall prevail.

Section B. Public Health

Professional responsibility demands that the optometrist actively participate in public health activities with other health professionals to the end that every step be taken to safeguard the health and welfare of the public.

The Optometric Oath

With full deliberation I freely and solemnly pledge that:

- I will practice the art and science of optometry faithfully and conscientiously, and to the fullest scope of my competence.

- I will uphold and honorably promote by example and action the highest standards, ethics and ideals of my chosen profession and the honor of the degree, Doctor of Optometry, which has been granted me.

- I will provide professional care for those who seek my services, with concern, with compassion and with due regard for their human rights and dignity.

- I will place the treatment of those who seek my care above personal gain and strive to see that none shall lack for proper care.

- I will hold as privileged and inviolable all information entrusted to me in confidence by my patients.

- I will advise my patients fully and honestly of all which may serve to restore, maintain or enhance their vision and general health.

- I will strive continuously to broaden my knowledge and skills so that my patients may benefit from all new and efficacious means to enhance the care of human vision.

- I will share information cordially and unselfishly with my fellow optometrists and other professionals for the benefit of patients and the advancement of human knowledge and welfare.

- I will do my utmost to serve my community, my country and humankind as a citizen as well as an optometrist.

I hereby commit myself to be steadfast in the performance of this my solemn oath and obligation.

References

1. Sanbar SS. A brief history of medical ethics. *Legal Med Persp* 1992; 1: 3-4.
2. Hippocrates. The oath. In: Chadwick J, Mann WN. *Hippocratic writings.* London: Penguin Books, 1978: 67.
3. Zaner RM. *Ethics and the clinical encounter.* Englewood Cliffs, NJ: Prentice Hall, 1988: 205-19.
4. Beauchamp TL, Walters LR. *Contemporary issues in bioethics*, 3rd ed. Belmont, CA: Wadsworth Publishing Co., 1989.
5. Bailey RN. The history of ethics in the American Optometric Association 1898-1994. *J Am Optom Assoc* 1994; 65: 427-44.
6. Code of ethics in final form. *J Am Optom Assoc* 1945 Jan; 16(6): 132-6.
7. American Optometric Association. Standards of conduct. St. Louis, MO: AOA, 1976; amended 1999.
8. American Optometric Association. The optometric oath. St. Louis, MO: AOA, 1986.
9. Bailey RN. Professional behavior and the optometric profession. *J Am Optom Assoc* 1997; 68: 693-8.
10. Flores A. *Professional ideals.* Belmont, CA: Wadsworth Publishing Co., 1988.

Chapter Two

Ethical Decision Making in Clinical Practice

Elizabeth Heitman, PhD
R. Norman Bailey, OD

Determining the right thing to do for patients in optometric practice is relatively straightforward most of the time. In-depth professional training and clinical experience in diagnosis and treatment give optometrists insight into the best ways to improve and protect their patients' eye and visual health. But while technical skill is vital to good patient care, serving patients' needs raises questions that extend beyond the technical realm of what *can* be done to the area of ethics and what *should* be done. A primary goal of this *Guide* is to lay out and discuss some of the more important ethical standards of clinical optometry as a baseline for practitioners to use in their own work.

No matter how comprehensive the available ethical guidelines, however, there will still be occasions when professionals face unfamiliar ethical questions raised by new technology or must resolve unexpected conflicts between principles or practice standards. In such instances, systematic methods of ethical reasoning and decision making are essential tools for clinical practice. Ethical analysis and decision making are skills that can be learned and which, when practiced, can become almost second nature for many clinicians. This chapter offers some perspectives on ethical decision making, presents a framework for considering ethical questions in clinical optometric practice, and discusses the use of the case method in teaching ethical analysis.

Ethics, Values, Principles, and Standards

The terms *ethics* and *morals** come respectively from the Greek and

---

* The terms ethics and morals, and ethical and moral, will be considered synonyms and used interchangeably throughout this book.

Latin words for *customs*, practices and rituals that are what ethicist Robert Bellah has called "the habits of the heart."[1] Although customs may appear to be superficial behaviors on one level, they often reflect a society's deepest, unconscious, sense of right and wrong. Ethics as a discipline is the study and analysis of values and standards related to duty, responsibility, and right and wrong behavior. Values are typically ideals that reflect the perceived worth of people, things, activities, and social institutions. Not all values are moral values; for example, both beauty and taste are esthetic rather than ethical values. Standards are typically stated expectations of performance, usually for a specific group or for a class of individuals.

The obligations that optometrists have toward their patients, each other, and society derive from ethical values held by both the optometric profession and by the larger community. Since the time of Hippocrates some of the more important moral values in health care have included trust, respect for life, benefiting others, avoiding harm to others, confidentiality, and collegiality. Both professional societies and governments have established standards for ethical practice that attempt to translate values into specific guides for professional behavior. The American Optometric Association (AOA) Code of Ethics, the AOA Standards of Conduct, and The Optometric Oath provide such guidance for practicing optometrists.

Contemporary bioethicists have also attempted to distill professional and societal values into formal theoretical principles that can be used for broad-based ethical analysis by individuals both inside and outside of the health care professions.[2] The most widely known set of ethical principles in health care includes: the principle of helping others (beneficence) and its corollary, doing no harm (nonmaleficence); respect for individuals' right to make their own choices (autonomy); and the fair distribution of goods and services and the need to treat similar cases similarly (justice). Other associated principles include truth telling and the avoidance of deception; respect for confidentiality and patients' need to reveal sensitive personal information during treatment; protection of the vulnerable, especially those who are unable to exercise autonomy; collegiality; and professional competence in practice.

Because these principles are easily recognized as being among the primary ethical goals of health care, using them as the basis for ethical analysis may help to explain the moral justification for certain professional actions, as well as to identify unethical behavior. However, in clinical practice, the specific demands and rationales of these broad principles may conflict. For example, the clinician's dedication to beneficence and nonmaleficence may be challenged when an autonomous patient refuses a recommended intervention. Similarly, the demands of justice may conflict with beneficence and respect for the patient's autonomy when the optometrist must decide how to fit in a walk-in patient with a significant problem when the appointment schedule is fully booked. In some situations where principles conflict, standards of practice and professional behavior may help define the right course of action. Nonetheless, because they are intended to be specific, professional standards may not apply well to situations that were not anticipated when the standards were laid out.

Whenever the optometrist faces a situation in which the best ethical course of action is unclear, such as when actions motivated by one ethical principle or standard conflict directly with other ethical principles or standards, it can be useful to analyze the situation in a structured way before acting. The goal of ethical decision making in clinical optometry should be to identify one or more courses of action that will honor the profession's essential values while minimizing conflict with other values and professional standards. Considering the relevant ethical issues formally may clarify the hierarchy of professional values related to the problem, and may identify a wider range of acceptable options than first seemed available.

At times, two or more mutually exclusive actions may appear to be supported by equally powerful moral arguments. This situation is known as a dilemma. Dilemmas by their very nature cannot be resolved by analytic methods — some ethical value must always be compromised. Fortunately, true ethical dilemmas are rare in optometry. Unfortunately, just as the very best optometric care may still have a poor outcome, even thoughtful ethical decision making may have tragic results for the patient, doctor, or both, due to unforeseen circumstances or incomplete information. Such cases are still useful to analyze if they can serve as lessons in the prevention of ethical conflict.

The process of ethical analysis and decision making outlined below can be adapted to fit the specific circumstances and needs of almost any optometrist and situation. While such analysis may be an almost instinctive part of clinical reasoning among experienced practitioners, there are few clinicians who cannot benefit from taking time for conscious reflection on factors that may be overlooked in the often emotionally charged setting of ethical conflict.

A Framework for Ethical Analysis and Decision Making

Step 1. *Recognize and identify the ethical problem(s).*

A stepwise process of ethical decision making begins with a comprehensive understanding of the problem. Remarkably, one of the hardest parts of ethical analysis is recognizing that a clinical problem involves a question of ethics. Many health care professionals are trained to see problems primarily in technical terms, and may believe that proper diagnosis and appropriate knowledge of treatment options are sufficient to define an acceptable course of action. Although ethical decision making is often portrayed as an unemotional, rational process, an unexpected negative emotional response to a situation is often an indication of an ethical problem. Anger, confusion, frustration, and even disgust can be signals that more careful analysis is called for.

Step 2. *Identify the clinically relevant facts, establish important definitions, and gather any additional necessary information.*

As in clinical diagnosis, it is important to have the essential facts of the situation before making a judgment. Some important questions to consider include:

- Who are the principal parties involved in the situation, what is their relationship, and what do they think are their respective roles?

- What are the relevant clinical, social, and financial facts of the matter? Which facts (if any) are in dispute? What information is missing?

■ How are the facts and definition of key concepts interpreted by the relevant parties? Why do they believe the problem exists? What do they think is the solution?

■ When did events important to the situation occur, and when does a decision need to be made to address the identified problems?

Seeking more information can frequently resolve many issues, and outside advice can be as helpful in clinical ethics as in other aspects of patient care. Conferring with others can provide new perspectives and new options. However, uncertainty about some aspects of the question may be unavoidable, and the problem is likely to need a response even when it is impossible to know basic related facts.

Step 3. *Identify relevant professional ethical codes, ethical practice standards, and ethical principles, and where conflict may exist between them.*

Although every patient encounter is unique, much about ethical patient care can be described in general terms. Determining whether the issue in question is addressed by the AOA, in either the Code of Ethics, the Standards of Conduct, or a resolution from the House of Delegates, may provide a starting point for consideration if not a definitive action plan. Similarly, relevant state and federal law may provide some general guides for action. (See Chapter 1 on the limited applicability of the law in ethical analysis.) If there is conflict between formal authoritative statements on the issue in question, consider the principles that the statements reflect, and whether there is any hierarchy among them. How do specific standards relate to other important values and standards; i.e., is any standard more important than others and why?

Step 4. *Identify the possible alternative courses of action and their likely outcomes.*

Considering the goals that are most important to achieve and the standards of behavior that are most important to follow, outline a best case, worst case, and middle ground scenario. Determine whether the means (the actions) or the ends (the outcomes) are more important ethically in this situation. It is important to recognize that the ideal scenario may not be possible to achieve, or possible only with significant sacrifice. Because some alternatives may create additional conflicts for various parties, tracing out the possible consequences of potential actions may prevent new problems from arising.

Step 5. *Choose the course that is best supported by your analysis and act accordingly.*

Not to act is to act by default. Health care professionals are held ethically accountable for the outcomes of patient care as well as for their specific actions, and it is professionally more responsible for the optometrist in a difficult situation to make a reasoned choice than to leave the problem to outside forces. In a litigious environment, many clinicians may be tempted to act against their professional judgment in response to the real or imagined demands of patients and insurers. However, it is ethically preferable and better risk management for practitioners to act in a way that 1) is consistent with good clinical practice, 2) is supported by a clear process of reasoning, and 3) they believe in personally. The rationale for such ethical decisions, as well as the consequent actions, should always be carefully documented in the patient's chart.

Step 6. *Evaluate the actions taken and their subsequent outcome.*

After acting upon a considered ethical decision, it is important to observe how closely what occurs matches what was predicted. By evaluating such actions and their outcomes, it may be possible to redirect events that do not go as expected, as well as to learn how similar decisions might work in the future. Conscious reflection on practice gives clinicians skill in ethical analysis and decision making, which can become an almost instinctive understanding of how to proceed when an ethical issue arises. Discussing such experiences with colleagues can also provide valuable feedback, including confirmation of professional standards of care. At the organizational level, communication with others about unusual clinical ethics issues can inform the profession about problems on the horizon, and permit the formulation of a policy response.

The Case Method in the Study of Ethics

The case method is an important tool in the study of ethics. Ethics courses in many health professions' training programs involve the analysis of classic cases as well as cases from faculty members' own professional experience. The case method relies on the presentation of a clinical scenario with sufficient detail to make it real but generalizable. Although case studies in ethics are increasingly available in textbooks and journals, an instructor's personal involvement in the case can be especially valuable in the information gathering stage (Step 2). Students' enthusiasm for discussion often increases when they know a case is "real," although it is essential for the presenter to omit names and change identifying details where the confidentiality of any party might be at stake.

After presenting a case, the instructor asks the group to identify the ethical question(s) it raises, *without* attempting to analyze them until a variety of questions have been spelled out. Important assumptions and biases are often revealed in the formulation of ethical questions, and their phrasing can be discussed as part of the later analysis. The instructor may also break questions into simpler components or add questions that others have not identified.

Questions may be discussed in the order in which they were raised, or in an order that appears to flow logically to the instructor. Discussion of each question should initially follow the first four steps for analysis, although after a few questions the relevant factual information and professional standards may already be established. After this discussion, the group should formulate a plan to address the issues that the case raises. In some cases, it may be possible to achieve consensus on the primary course of action, but in others not. In both situations, the group should consider how to evaluate the consequences of their decision, and what events might make them change their minds.

Each of the following chapters includes a clinical case that illustrates different aspects of their respective topics. These cases are fictitious, although based in the authors' professional experience, and are offered as examples of scenarios that might arise in clinical practice in many settings.‡ We suggest that you examine the case both before and after reading the chapter, and compare your perspectives and preferred course of action. As this *Guide* is intended to be useful as a textbook as well as reference for optometrists already in practice, we encourage the use of these cases in formal teaching as well as formal and informal professional discussion.

References

1. Bellah R. *Habits of the heart*. New York: Harper Collins, 1996.
2. Beauchamp T, Childress J. *Principles of biomedical ethics*, 4th ed. New York: Oxford University Press, 1994.

---

‡ The cases presented here were written specifically for inclusion in this volume. Any similarity between the circumstances or characters described in these cases and actual events involving actual persons, living or dead, is purely coincidental.

Chapter Three

Communicating with Patients in the Doctor-Patient Relationship

R. Norman Bailey, OD
Elizabeth Heitman, PhD

Dr. Wilson had just completed his examination of elderly Mrs. Dobbs' eyes and vision and had determined that she had advanced diabetic retinopathy in the periphery of both eyes. He was preparing to discuss his diagnostic findings with her when she advised him, "whatever you have found, I do not want you to tell my daughter, she would just worry too much…and if it is anything serious requiring surgery, I do not want to know anything about it. I have lived a long life and I don't want to spend the last of it having to deal with lots of complicated medical procedures."

At least as long ago as the writing of the Hippocratic Oath, it was well understood that physicians' communication with their patients was an essential part of successful therapy. The relationship between a doctor and patient should be based upon trust, which develops mainly through communication. In much of health care, accurate diagnosis and appropriate treatment depend upon the patient's truthful and complete disclosure of personal health information. For a trusting therapeutic relationship to be established and maintained, patients need to know that their doctor will keep their personal information confidential, and use it only to help them. Doctors, likewise, need to know that their patients will be forthcoming about their histories, symptoms, and goals of treatment, and honest about following agreed-upon therapies.

From the Hippocratic era until early this century, doctors had few real treatments for most conditions, and they recognized that their most effective therapy was their simple reassurance that the patient was going to get better. Using what we today recognize as the power of the placebo effect, doctors consciously promoted patients' hope for recovery through their

19

controlled communication of diagnostic and prognostic information. This strategy reflected the belief common to both doctors and patients that the doctor should withhold diagnostic and prognostic information that might make the patient depressed or give up hope. Until the latter part of this century, doctors' communication with patients often involved deception and the withholding of "bad news" in an effort to create hope and maintain therapeutic trust.

Since at least the 1970s, the practice of deception and withholding information in health care has been widely condemned by patients, ethicists, and clinicians. Because today's patients are often concerned about maintaining their own health and well educated about health-related issues in general, they both want and understand meaningful information from their health care providers. The patient's rights movement of the last three decades has emphasized that patients have a right to make their own health care decisions based on a full understanding of their options. While clinicians still recognize the importance of good communication in building therapeutic trust, this trust is now believed to be based in the doctor's truthfulness and respect for the patient's autonomy. Today truth telling and informed consent, rather than deceptive reassurance, are the standard for good clinical communication.

Communication and Informed Consent

Informed consent serves the vital purpose of strengthening patients' participation in and control over their health care. The ethical principle behind informed consent is respect for patient autonomy. The term autonomy has its root in ancient Greek and means self-rule or self-determination. Where the goal of communication with patients is to protect their right to self-determination and enhance their participation in their own eye and vision care, optometrists must be aware of the standards of behavior that support this end.

Open communication with patients is essential to identifying and removing barriers that may interfere with their ability to participate fully in and maintain some control over their care. U.S. society has deemed a patient's right to self-determination so important that every state has informed consent laws that define the information that clinicians must give to patients when they recommend a specific intervention. These laws are based on the premise that, before they can participate fully in decisions about any diagnostic or therapeutic procedure, patients must have enough information to make an informed choice. In the standard process of informed consent, the patient must be told about 1) the diagnosis or problem to be addressed; 2) the proposed intervention; 3) the risks and benefits of the proposed intervention; and 4) any alternatives to the proposed intervention — including doing nothing — and their risks and benefits.

The extent of the information that must be provided in a particular case varies according to the degree of intervention required and the attendant risks of the procedure. The more complex the procedure or greater the risk, the more formal the disclosure and consent process must be. The spectrum of informed consent ranges from *implied* consent to a "routine" examination, in which the patient's presenting for an appointment implies the patient's willingness to be examined, to *simple consent* to a low-risk procedure after the patient receives basic information about the intervention, to *written informed consent* following the disclosure of comprehensive information and the formal signing of a consent document prior to the procedure.[1] Under even the best of conditions, however, patients still have less knowledge and ability than the optometrist to understand the recommended procedure and, therefore, must trust the optometrist's commitment to act in their best interest.

While informed consent law is very important in protecting patients' rights to self-determination, the process of informed consent can be complicated by a number of factors. The paternalistic assumption that the doctor knows best, and that the patient should simply "follow the doctor's orders," has been discredited only in the last generation, and many optometrists as well as patients are uncomfortable with a more egalitarian partnership. Optometrists bring a knowledge base and professional vocabulary to clinical discussion that are largely foreign to lay people, and which give them significant power over their patients. Even where the optometrist promotes good communication, patients are frequently inhibited in their participation by uncertainty, fear, denial, coercion, economic interests, and cultural characteristics.[2] They bring to the discussion personal experiences and beliefs related to their conditions that the optometrist may not fully understand.

The ability to listen carefully to patients is an important clinical skill in optometry. In disclosing diagnostic information and treatment options, the optometrist must recognize the patient's concerns, and be mindful of the assumptions underlying the patient's words as well as unspoken messages that may be conveyed in body language. When the situation is emotionally charged, as in the case of Dr. Wilson and Mrs. Dobbs, the potential for incomplete communication or miscommunication is great. The informed consent process may be clouded by the patient's fear of disease or disability, as well as anxiety about the demands of possible treatment.

Some patients fear making the "wrong" decision about their care, and hesitate to choose among alternative treatment options when they are uncertain about the acceptability of the outcome. Their uncertainty may range from concern about financial risk, to changes in their appearance, to losing all vision. Some want "doctor's orders" that relieve them of personal responsibility for the outcome of their choices, and in the face of uncertainty may state outright, "You're the doctor, you tell me what I should do." Additional discussion of the risks and benefits of each option, or a second opinion, may help such patients, but some may be frustrated when the optometrist can give them no guarantee. The optometrist's general willingness to make choices for hesitant patients may create difficulties when such decisions result in unfavorable outcomes. At the least, the dissatisfied patient may blame the optometrist for the negative outcome; unfortunately this dissatisfaction may result in malpractice litigation that claims the optometrist usurped the patient's right to informed consent.

Patients like Mrs. Dobbs may refuse diagnostic information or deny that they have a significant health problem in the face of overwhelming evidence. At times, patients may refuse to discuss any diagnosis that implies a loss of independence. Such denial is often a psychological response to the fear of blindness, and the fear of losing the ability to choose may be greater than the fear of death.[3] Patients may be particularly affected by denial in the early stages of chronic conditions when no symptoms are present, as in the case of glaucoma and early diabetic retinopathy. It is often difficult to get patients to consider treatment for these and other chronic ocular conditions. In such cases, patient education is essential, and the optometrist may have an ethical responsibility to obtain a second opinion or introduce the patient to relevant support groups.

Whenever fear appears to limit the patient's abilities to participate in treatment decisions, it is essential that the optometrist assess the source of that fear and help the patient to assume greater responsibility for his or her health care. Because of the potential ambiguity of indirect and nonverbal communication, the optometrist may need to verify his or her perceptions by addressing them directly. Then, too, the optometrist's choice of words and tone of voice become very important in preventing the creation of new, baseless fears for patients who are intimidated by the technical nature of the discussion. Patients who are emotionally unprepared to hear bad news may be unable to understand what the optometrist says in even the simplest language.

In many circumstances, the simple communication required under informed consent law is only a minimum disclosure that does not meet the ethical standard of involving the patient actively in the decision-making process. The disparity in clinical knowledge between them often makes the patient dependent upon the optometrist to interpret the information as well as to disclose it. Through good communication the optometrist can reduce the gap by describing not only the reasonable options available to the patient, but also why one option may be preferable to the others in the patient's particular circumstances. In the ethical ideal of informed consent, the optometrist's thought processes should become "transparent" to the patient.[4] Such transparency helps the optometrist avoid deliberate or subconscious coercion of the patient to simply accept a single recommended treatment. Patients who understand the reasoning behind the options that the optometrist presents can make treatment decisions with confidence both in their own judgment and in the optometrist who will treat them.

In contrast, nothing is likely to interfere more with the trust between patient and doctor than the patient's perception that the doctor has a significant personal interest in a specific treatment. Of particular concern is the conflict of interest that may occur when the optometrist stands to benefit financially or professionally from one particular treatment option. Whether such benefit is related to rebates from the ophthalmic industry, enhanced earnings from using the newest hot technology, or professional enhancement from participating in a clinical research project, optometrists must carefully analyze the impact that any potential financial or professional gain may have upon the advice they give to their patients. In addition, in compliance with any applicable laws, the financial or professional benefit to the practitioner should be revealed to the patient when it is directly related to the recommendation.

Beyond the positive effects of creating trust, the optometrist's effective communication with patients is also essential for the successful outcomes of many, if not most, treatments. A patient who does not fully understand the recommended plan of treatment may have difficulty following it, and without adherence to plan, the desired treatment outcome may not be achieved. In this context, too, the Hippocratic teachings about the effects of reassurance are still quite valid: compassionate and supportive communication about treatment can itself be therapeutic. Implicit in the process of informed consent is the optometrist's ethical responsibility to reassure patients that, whatever the outcome of their condition or treatment, they will not be abandoned.[5]

Surrogate Consent and Confidentiality

Some patients are more capable than others of making reasonable health care decisions. The law presumes that adults are competent to make their own medical decisions unless a judge has determined that they are mentally or physically unable to act in their own best interests. When an individual is declared incompetent, a guardian is appointed to make his or her decisions regarding important issues such as health care. Children and adolescents are presumed to be incompetent by virtue of their minor age, and their parents or guardians are typically responsible for health care decision on their behalf. Although such surrogate decision makers give formal consent for treatment, even incompetent patients should be included in discussion of their care to the extent that they have the capacity to understand and assent to treatment.

Most practices include a number of patients who have no legal guardian but who may be assisted in making treatment decisions by family members or other surrogate decision makers. Sometimes these patients are unable to participate fully in the informed consent process and communication about their care for reasons of limited or impaired mental capacity or other disabling conditions. Others simply seem to need the support of family or friends. However, support for the patient must be tempered by concern for the patient's privacy and confidentiality. Little is more private to patients than discussions surrounding their health. Like Mrs. Dobbs, some patients may not want family members to know important information about their conditions, and they have the right to determine who has access to even the most trivial information.

The protection of patient confidentiality is another ancient ethical duty, dating from the fourth century BCE, when the Hippocratic Oath proclaimed that "whatever I see or hear, professionally or privately, which ought not to be divulged, I will keep secret and tell no one."[6] Keeping patient information confidential probably contributes as much as any other ethical standard or conduct to the trust that holds the doctor-patient relationship together. This is true at all levels of health care, from highly specialized services to the general care provided by the family optometrist.

When a patient is accompanied to an appointment by family members or friends, it is essential for the optometrist to determine what role such persons are meant to have in the patient's treatment before they are included in any discussion of the patient's condition. Often this means that the optometrist must talk to the patient alone for at least long enough to ask who else is authorized to take part in the conversation. In this way, too, the optometrist may learn important information about the patient's support system that may help promote later adherence to recommended treatment. In situations where the patient will likely need assistance dealing with a diagnosis or treatment plan, as in the case of Mrs. Dobbs, the optometrist can offer to help the patient talk with family members rather than leaving difficult conversations to the patient alone.

One particularly important challenge for optometrists across the United States is the rising number of immigrants with limited English language skills. Significant cultural differences make good communication more important, but also more difficult as real dialogue is typically impossible without an interpreter.[7] Because many non-English speaking patients are accompanied by family members with greater fluency in English, there is a great temptation to use these third parties to translate the interaction between the patient and the optometrist. Not only can this practice pose a real risk to patient confidentiality, it may also compromise communication. Unless the optometrist can verify the translator's knowledge of both English and the patient's language, there is no assurance that information will be conveyed accurately. Moreover, patients may lie or withhold information rather than reveal sensitive information to family members, and family members may provide their own views rather than translating questions or comments. As is discussed in Chapter 14, whenever possible, optometrists in areas with significant non-English speaking populations should have bi-lingual staff or access to high-quality interpreting to ensure the best care for their patients.

Finally, in addition to communication in the clinical setting, it is impor-tant to take care in managing both paper and electronic records to protect patients' rights to privacy. Third-party participation in the care of patients often involves sharing records and clinical information with others, such as employers, that the patient does not know have access to personal data. The most personal information is sometimes treated as though it were in the public domain. Optometrists should be diligent in safeguarding the trust of their patients in the confidentiality of personal disclosures, and when pos-sible, should avoid providing more information to third parties than is specifically requested.

References

1. Abplanalp P. Informed consent as an ethical issue in modern optometry. *J Am Optom Assoc* 1994; 65: 347-54.
2. Bailey RN. The doctor-patient relationship: communication, informed consent and the optometric patient. *J Am Optom Assoc* 1994; 65: 418-22.
3. Zaner RM. *Ethics and the clinical encounter*. Englewood Cliffs, NJ: Prentice Hall, 1988, 266-82.

4. Brody H. Transparency: informed consent in primary care. *Hastings Center Rept* 1989; 19(Sep/Oct): 5-9.
5. Katz J. *The silent world of doctor and patient.* New York: Free Press, 1984.
6. Hippocrates. The oath. In: Chadwick J, Mann WN, trans. *Hippocratic writings.* London: Penguin Books, 1978, 267.
7. Heitman E. Cultural diversity and the clinical encounter: intercultural dialogue in multi-ethnic patient care. In: McKenny GP, Sande JR, eds. *Theological analyses of the clinical encounter.* New York: Reidel, 1994, 203-23.

Chapter Four

Shared Responsibility in Patient Care

Brian S. Klinger, OD

Returning from a quick lunch, Dr. Casey, a busy solo practitioner, goes over her phone messages with the receptionist. The receptionist reports that Mr. Salisbury had called, asking for an immediate appointment in what already looks like a hectic afternoon. The receptionist relates that, following Dr. Casey's triage instructions, she asked Mr. Salisbury whether he was in pain and what kind of symptoms he was having. "He said that he was sorry to be calling right before his annual exam, but that he just broke his only glasses, and that his right eye is sort of red and swollen. I was going to have him come in right away. But then I checked his record to see about his glasses — he's a 4 diopter myope — and I saw that last year's exam notes said that he called in two weeks before his scheduled appointment with a very similar story about a red eye. You saw him right away, but his eyes were fine. I think he's just trying to get a more convenient appointment. I told him you were very busy today and gave him an appointment tomorrow when we have a little more room in the schedule. Do you want to talk to him?"

Certain questions are unique to an office practice, where the principal doctor is the proprietor, as compared with a hospital-based or large-clinic setting. The optometrist who provides most of the patient care in an office practice frequently is the owner of both the professional practice and the associated optical dispensary, and thus may be the employer of a variety of professional, technical, and clerical staff. The assistance of staff members is essential to running any practice. As an employer, owner, and professional caregiver, the optometrist must ensure that staff members understand and fulfill their individual and shared responsibilities to the practice and its patients.[1,2] Even a receptionist's overbooking, so that the optometrist is chronically behind schedule, creates ethical conflicts that the optometrist is ultimately responsible to prevent.

29

Distinguishing Roles and Responsibilities in the Office Setting

Optometrists have a duty to their patients and staff, as well as to their profession, to make sure that everyone in the office knows that the patient's welfare will always be of uppermost importance. Staff members, in return, have a duty to the optometrist to support the ethical standards of the practice. In general, the optometrist in charge of the practice must be aware that even long-time patients may not "know the ropes," and that they have to trust the staff to look out for their interests just as they expect the optometrist to do. This means that, if the best care is to be rendered, it is the optometrist's obligation to make the office as "user-friendly" as possible. The doctor must make sure that the staff is properly trained to deal with patients. All staff need to have good telephone and face-to-face communication skills, know how to maintain patients' confidentiality, and know when to seek the optometrist's direct involvement in a problem that arises in their work.[3] Regular training and evaluation can ensure that every staff member knows how to act so that the patient's needs are served at all times.

Little practical things, such as requiring personnel to wear name tags so the patients know who is who, and having the caregivers and technicians wear different uniforms, really reflect ethical concern for the patients' trust and confidence in the practice. Just as the common hospital dress code that allows everyone to wear scrubs makes it hard to distinguish among doctors, nurses, technicians, and the cleaning staff, optometrists must be aware of behaviors that unfairly force patients to guess who is responsible for what part of their care. When situations arise where the patient has direct contact only with a staff member rather than with the optometrist, the staff member must be able to explain his or her role in the patient's care. Patients accustomed to seeing the optometrist at every visit may also need reassurance about the staff member's qualifications and the optometrist's ultimate oversight of what is done.

Nonetheless, it is important that the optometrist be able to rely on staff and employees to make judgments that will affect the welfare of patients. Often this means providing staff with guidelines on what is expected of them in predictable circumstances, such as "emergency" calls. In turn, the staff has a responsibility to the optometrist to follow these guidelines, to explain them to patients as necessary, and to report to the optometrist situations in which they cannot apply the guidelines without creating new problems.

Calls from patients like Mr. Salisbury are an almost daily occurrence in a successful office practice. The ethical question raised by his request for an immediate appointment with Dr. Casey can be summarized as how to weigh the right of already-scheduled patients to receive enough of the doctor's (and the staff members') time to ensure adequate care, against the right of another patient to timely attention in what he or she perceives to be an urgent or emergent situation. Unless the situation is truly urgent, the doctor owes a greater duty to the patients already booked. If there is no urgency in a patient's request for an immediate appointment, the optometrist must not shortchange other previously booked patients by making them wait longer than truly necessary. "Squeezing in" another examination might serve the doctor's interests by placating one patient, but would not serve the other patients' interests at all. Conversely, no one would disagree that a patient in pain or with a potentially serious set of symptoms should be seen right away.

In such circumstances, it is essential for the staff member responsible for scheduling to be able to distinguish between an emergency and non-emergency situation, to know when to ask the optometrist for a more in-depth assessment of the patient's request to be seen, and to determine how best to fit the unexpected patient into the schedule. Additionally, he or she may need to be able to explain the nature of the emergency to other patients who may be inconvenienced by the emergency visit, and offer them appropriate alternative scheduling if they need it. Moreover, if the doctor sincerely tries to take care of every patient as fully as possible, staff and employees may also need to be willing to work extra hours to get back on schedule and avoid keeping patients waiting long past their scheduled appointment times.

Conflicts of Interest and Staff Members' Responsibilities in Patient Care

Optometrists must be aware that they may face conflicts of interest between the financial welfare of their practice and the actual needs of their patients. For many optometrists, the more patients seen, the more services, tests, and procedures rendered to the patient, and the more eyeglasses, frames, and contact lenses sold through the dispensary, the greater the practice's profit will be. On the other hand, a patient's best interest may not be best served by an extra test performed, an extra visit scheduled, an extra pair of glasses recommended, or an extra prescription change. The potential for such conflicts of interests exists in any practice setting, but the office practice is more vulnerable to the temptations generated by the direct profit motive than are practitioners in a large clinic or hospital where profit does not go directly to the doctor.

Fewer optometrists recognize that the potential for such conflicts also extends to the practice's staff. For example, paying bonuses or commission to staff based on the dollar volume of the dispensary may encourage them to "push" unnecessary accessories and multiple pairs of eyeglasses. Just as the optometrist should assess the real need for every prescription, staff should make only those recommendations that they would if the patient were filling the prescription at another dispensary. Still, even without direct financial incentives to them, staff or employees may sometimes act in ways that they think will help the optometrist or the practice in general, but which are not in the patient's best interest. Because most staff may not fully appreciate the essential ethical commitments of the health care professions, it is often easier for them to recognize the business-oriented goals of the practice. Thus it is the optometrist's responsibility to distinguish clearly between the standards of ethical patient care and the standards of good business as they affect each employee's work.[4]

In an office practice, the actions of the staff may also create conflicts of interest for the optometrist more directly than in other settings, since they may be given more responsibility than they would be in similar positions in a larger facility. Optometrists who give their staff greater responsibility for patient care must ensure that their employees have sufficient ethical awareness to carry out these responsibilities, and that the staff knows that they are accountable to the optometrist for decisions that affect patients' welfare. For example, although Dr. Casey clearly relied on her receptionist for scheduling and triage, the receptionist did the right thing in bringing Mr. Salisbury's situation to her attention. If the receptionist had simply told Mr. Salisbury to come in the next day, without telling Dr. Casey about the patient's call or her rationale for rescheduling him, the optometrist would not have known about the patient's possible infection until after treatment had been delayed. As this case demonstrates, it is essential for staff to know the limits of their knowledge and authority, and to know when to turn to the optometrist with questions.

Continuity of Care

The need for continuity of care is another issue in which the optometrist's duty to patients may require sharing responsibility for patients with others, and which likely requires having a formal plan in place. An optometrist who thinks that his or her responsibility to patients ends at 5 PM is mistaken, both ethically and legally. Ensuring continuity of care clearly means that there must be some system in place for after-hours coverage for emergencies. A system that allows a patient to contact a qualified practitioner after hours in an emergency meets the ethical test for availability; a voice on an answering machine stating that the office will be open again in the morning does not.

When a practice has more than one optometrist, whether in a small office or in a larger clinic, it is likely that more than one will see the same patients over time. After as little as one visit patients often recognize one optometrist as their eye doctor, and may expect to be treated by someone familiar at all future visits. Whereas it is important to respect and support the patient's good relationship with a particular optometrist, it is not always possible to honor a patient's request to be seen by a specific caregiver in a multi-person office. The possibility of being treated by any of the practice's optometrists is most easily conveyed to new patients just learning about the operation of the office. When a patient must be seen by an unfamiliar caregiver, it is important for the staff member who schedules the appointment to tell the patient which optometrist will provide the examination or treatment. It may also be necessary to assure the patient that such cross-coverage is a normal activity of the practice. The optometrist who treats a colleague's patient may similarly need to reassure the patient that his or her original optometrist will still be in charge of the case.

Providing continuity of care through cross-coverage within a practice raises two important ethical issues: fairness in dealing with colleagues, and providing the best care to patients. In most situations, the primary means of communicating about patients' treatment by different caregivers is through the patient record. If more than one optometrist will be likely to see the same patient, it is essential for everyone to be sure that their records are complete and legible so that colleagues can readily establish an unfamiliar patient's diagnostic and treatment history. The use of jargon, abbreviations, and personal shorthand should be avoided in patient records, as they may be misinterpreted and put the patient at risk of harm. Even in a single-practitioner office this should always be the standard for record keeping, for no one can predict when illness or an accident might necessitate bringing another optometrist into the practice temporarily.

Additional issues may arise from optometrists' need to share clinical responsibilities in a growing practice, as in the common situation where a young doctor is taken on as an associate or junior partner. How the junior colleague will establish a patient base may be problematic. Should the new partner take on all the patients the senior colleague does not want, such as the indigent patients, the chronic complainers, and those who are lacking in personal hygiene? Unless the plan had been made clear during the employment or contract negotiation process, such "dumping" would violate the principle of fairness toward both the new optometrist and to the patients who may have wanted to stay with the senior clinician. On the other hand, a well-intentioned attempt to keep the young doctor's schedule booked that resulted in scheduling some "difficult" established patients would not be unfair. Of course, if the younger optometrist has special skills or advanced training in a particular area, a transfer would be equally advantageous to patients with related special needs, the new optometrist, and the practice as a whole.

Shared Responsibility in Referral

Every optometrist has a duty to provide the best possible care to any patient he or she undertakes to treat. Many times all necessary care can be rendered in the office, but the optometrist has a responsibility to recognize that some patients may need to be seen by others outside of the practice. For example, when either the optometrist is in doubt about the patient's diagnosis, or when the patient is not responding as expected to the prescribed treatment, the patient would likely benefit from a referral for a second opinion. The optometrist in such circumstances has a responsibility to suggest that a second opinion would be desirable and to recommend a qualified colleague to provide it. If the patient accepts the recommendation, the original optometrist must provide complete and useful clinical information to the colleague, who should render the requested opinion promptly, in writing, and in language that does not disparage the original optometrist's need for a second opinion.[5]

Occasionally, a patient may feel more comfortable with the second optometrist than with the original clinician who arranged for the visit. In some cases the patient may directly express a wish to transfer all of his or her eye and vision care to the second optometrist. Although the patient's wishes must ultimately govern such a decision, both the original optometrist and the consultant should inform the patient from the outset that they are working together for the patient's best interest, and that the consultant is not intended as a replacement. The referring optometrist should make clear, and the consultant should clearly understand, that the patient is intended to return, and that the original optometrist remains responsible for the patient's comprehensive eye and vision care.

As is discussed in Chapter 5, a different dynamic comes into play when the patient's optometrist diagnoses a condition that is outside of his or her area of competence. For example, a patient whom the optometrist knows would benefit more from vision training than from glasses would need to be transferred, perhaps permanently, if that service is not offered in the practice. While there might be a temptation for the optometrist to keep the patient, and perhaps rationalize that choice with the argument that there is no assurance that the vision training would, in fact, be beneficial, the optometrist's responsibility to serving the patient's interests first requires that the patient should be advised of the potentially better course of treatment available elsewhere.

Optometrists' and Payers' Responsibilities to Patients

In recent years, as third-party payment has become common for a higher percentage of office patients, defining the optometrist's responsibilities to patients in light of restrictions imposed by payers has become a pressing problem. Consider the situation where an optometrist determines that a patient needs a drug that is not on the managed care organization's "approved" formulary list, or that a patient needs to be seen on a more frequent schedule than the plan will cover. In each case the insurers define their responsibility to cover care at a much lower level than the optometrist believes is necessary for the welfare of the patient. Where the optometrist has a formal contract with an insurer or managed care organization, the optometrist may be required to agree to a standard pre-set definition of appropriate treatment as the basis for payment or reimbursement for optometric services. In such cases, the optometrists' responsibilities to the insurer for cost-containment may conflict directly with the responsibility to serve the patient's best interests.

Like many of the ethical issues that optometrists face, there may not be a clear answer to the problem of such conflicting responsibilities. Should the doctor ever prescribe a course of treatment that is less than optimal because it is all that the insurer will pay for? Is a generic formulation an acceptable alternative to the better but more expensive brand-name drug? Are glasses a suitable option for a patient whose plan does not cover vision therapy? Certainly the first step to resolving these conflicts is to have a full and frank discussion with the patient about the payer's limits and why the optometrist believes the approved treatment to be inappropriate for the patient. It is ultimately the patient's choice to select the level of care that he or she wants and is willing and able to pay for apart from third-party coverage. Few patients with insurance or managed care coverage understand their eye and vision care benefits, and an informed decision must be based on facts as well as the advice of the doctor. In many such cases, the optometrist's responsibility to patients includes careful discussion of how and why the optometrist defines appropriate treatment differently from the patient's insurer.

An essential ethical principle of health care is that of "do no harm." In a situation where the optometrist believes that anything other than a specific course of treatment will cause the patient's condition to worsen, he or she must use every effort to convince the patient that the recommended intervention is essential — an offer to obtain a second opinion, written educational materials, discussions with other family members, etc. Moreover, the optometrist should make a concerted attempt to convince the insurer of the importance of paying for the disallowed intervention. Certainly, if the final choice is not the "best" drug or course of treatment, there needs to be full documentation of the decision and its rationale in the chart.

Every profession, every practice, and every practitioner is governed by not only legal constraints, but also by the ethical concerns of making sure that the patient is properly served. Considering our practices from a patient's perspective can help optometrists understand the multiple responsibilities of clinical practice. The "golden rule" of treating others as we would wish to be treated should be kept in mind constantly, and will help us render the kind of care we would wish to receive in a colleague's office.

References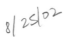

1. Rumpakis JM. Promoting teamwork. *Optom Manag* 1998; 33(8): 58-60.
2. Lakin DH, Rounds RS, Shaw McMinn P, Hisaka C. Managing an office staff. In: Classé JG, et al., eds., *Business aspects of optometry*. Boston, MA: Butterworth-Heinemann, 1997: 163-75.
3. Rothman S, Kaplan H, Hisaka C. Patient communication. In: Classé JG, et al., eds., *Business aspects of optometry*. Boston, MA: Butterworth-Heinemann, 1997: 177-85.
4. American Optometric Association. Resolution 1886, adopted 1991; modified 1995. AOA House of Delegates Resolutions and Substantive Motions. Judicial Council. St. Louis, MO: AOA, 1999.
5. Bridwell J, Usdan M, Farkas P. Interpersonal relations. In: Classé JG, et al., eds., *Business aspects of optometry*. Boston, MA: Butterworth-Heinemann, 1997: 187-96.

Chapter Five

Standards of Care and Collegial Relations

Thomas F. Dorrity, Jr., OD
R. Norman Bailey, OD

A long-time patient of Dr. Cartwright, Mrs. Johnson, has come in for a comprehensive eye and vision examination. Mrs. Johnson was diagnosed with Type II (non-insulin dependent) diabetes mellitus approximately two years ago. She reports that her diabetes is under control with oral medications and dietary restrictions. The standard of care calls for a yearly dilated fundus examination for all diabetic patients. Dr. Cartwright is 64 years old and plans to retire at the end of the year. Due to his approaching retirement, he has not bothered to obtain his state board's certification to use diagnostic or therapeutic pharmaceuticals. Rather than refer this long-time patient for dilation and admit to her that he is no longer able to provide the full scope of optometric care, he is considering just providing his usual direct ophthalmoscopy, and referring her for further evaluation only if he observes diabetic retinopathy in the posterior pole.

Providing high-level eye and vision care is the responsibility of both individual optometrists and the profession at large. Collegial interaction is essential to the sound practice of the individual optometrist. Individual practitioners have a responsibility to each other and to the public to advance the profession's knowledge base and recognize and address questionable practices in the field. Mutual accountability among members is a hallmark of professional integrity, and is one basis for the relative self-governance that society permits the professions in general.

The American Optometric Association (AOA) has repeatedly emphasized the importance of informed and competent practitioners working for the best interests of their patients. The AOA's Code of Ethics instructs optometrists to keep the visual welfare of patients uppermost at all times, to enhance continuously their education and technical proficiencies to the end that patients shall receive the benefits of all acknowledged improvements in visual care, and to conduct themselves as exemplary citizens.[1] The AOA's House of Delegates has adopted a number of related resolutions that specifically address the establishment and role of standards of care, the nature of professional relationships among practitioners, and the optometrist's responsibilities to colleagues who may not meet professional standards of practice because of impairment.[2]

Standards of Practice

Standards for patient care in optometry are shaped by a number of factors. Legal standards may be defined by state statute or by regulations promulgated by state boards of optometry. Differences in state legislation across the United States mean that it is possible for legislatively defined standards of care to vary from state to state. Legal standards also may be established in case law by courts of various jurisdictions. Malpractice litigation often turns on questions of standards of care, which are typically defined by expert witnesses rather than regulations alone.

Historically, courts accepted definitions of standards of care based on the practices accepted in the local community. However, in the past few decades, most states have abandoned the notion of local standards of practice in favor of national or universal standards.[3] Moreover, due to similarities in eye care provided by physicians and optometrists, standards defined by court decisions involving physicians are likely to be applied to optometrists providing the same type of service.[3] For example, in *Helling v. Carey*, a case involving an ophthalmologist, the state Supreme Court of Washington held that failure to test for glaucoma as part of a comprehensive eye examination is negligence as a matter of law.[4] This decision impacted the standard for tonometric examinations conducted by both ophthalmologists and optometrists across the nation.

Professional associations also help to establish standards of care. The AOA has published a number of Optometric Clinical Practice Guidelines covering various aspects of patient care.[5] Although these Guidelines are not legally binding, they are consensus documents that reflect the professional opinion of leaders in the field in the area of practice that they address. In addition, the House of Delegates of the AOA has adopted a number of resolutions recommending standards for optometric practice, many of which are based on formal research as well as policy debate.[2] Resolution 1924, "Maintaining High Standards for Eye and Vision Care," adopted in 1997, states specifically that, as a matter of ethical concern, optometrists should maintain the high standards of eye and vision care as set forth in the AOA's Optometric Clinical Practice Guidelines.*

Insurers, and particularly managed care organizations (MCOs), are another important source of standards of care. Insurers typically establish treatment protocols and definitions of medically necessary treatment as part of their contracts with practitioners. These standards reflect decisions about a treatment's relative cost-effectiveness as well as what are considered to be "best practices," and these insurers' standards may impact many optometrists' decisions.

Finally, organizations dedicated to research on and prevention and treatment of specific diseases may encourage health care providers to provide certain levels of care. For example, the American Diabetes Association includes guidelines on screening for diabetic retinopathy in its comprehensive recommendations on the medical care of persons with diabetes.[6] Guidelines promoted by disease advocacy groups may call for higher levels of care than standards developed by others, but they are usually backed by research that demonstrates the benefits of more intervention for their particular constituencies, and they offer an additional benchmark for practitioners and patients.

Ideally, the motive for defining standards of care, and the best reason for professionals to adhere to such standards, is the health benefits that

---

* Each of the Guidelines notes that, "Clinicians should not rely on this Clinical Guideline alone for patient care and management. Refer to the listed references and other sources for a more detailed analysis and discussion of research and patient care information. The information in the Guideline is current as of the date of publication. It will be reviewed periodically and revised as needed." AOA members may view on-line the entire text of each Clinical Practice Guideline on the AOA Member Website at www.aoanet.org/members/.

conforming to standards provides to patients. Establishing and following good practice standards acknowledges the ethical principle of beneficence. This ethical imperative is so compelling that society has granted an almost regulatory authority to many formal standards of practice. However, meeting the "legal standard" of care may not fulfill the ethical demands in a given clinical situation: often the legal standard is only a minimum that the practitioner must achieve.

Ethical issues may arise when practice standards appear to be motivated by factors other than patients' welfare. For example, treatment protocols and standards of care set by some MCOs may appear to be more profit oriented than patient oriented. Such standards often raise concern when their use attempts to limit or replace the optometrist's professional judgment in order to avoid the expense of more comprehensive or costly treatment. The optometrist's ethical duty demands that the patient's specific needs, as defined by sound clinical judgment, take priority over the demands of generalized standards or profit issues. Economic factors should be secondary to providing what is necessary to restore the patient to good ocular and visual health. Optometrists should be familiar with the practice guidelines issued by the insurers and the MCOs with which they work, and prepared with a plan of action in the event that their professional judgment calls for treatment that the plan will not approve.

Meeting the standard of care for some conditions often requires collegial collaboration and referral of patients with complex conditions. For example, as described in the case of Dr. Cartwright above, the AOA's *Optometric Clinical Practice Guideline for Care of the Patient with Diabetes Mellitus* recommends that diabetic patients receive a dilated fundus examination annually, with semiannual examinations for those patients with diabetic retinopathy. Doctors who do not practice the full scope of optometry have the ethical duty to refer patients at risk for diabetic eye disease to a practitioner who is able to carry out the necessary procedures. Even when an optometrist is qualified to diagnose certain conditions or undertake technical procedures, in some cases consultation with a more experienced or specialized practitioner may benefit the patient. Moreover, optometrists who recognize signs of non-ophthalmic diseases in an undiagnosed patient have a duty to refer the patient to a physician for a more comprehensive medical evaluation.

Collegial Relations

The process of referral and consultation may raise a number of ethical issues of collegial relations. Some optometrists may hesitate to seek assistance from another practitioner for fear of not appearing competent to either their patient or their colleague. Others may believe that, whatever their own limits, no other practitioner can provide comparable care. Others may worry that a request for short-term collegial assistance may result in the permanent loss of a patient, beyond the reason for the referral.

Patients have a right to expect the proper referral when their condition warrants, as well as a right to a full explanation of the need for the second opinion and/or treatment from another practitioner. Similarly, the referring optometrist must explain to the consultant the reasons for the referral and the nature of the needed work. Failing to share relevant information, whether related to the original optometrists' limits or the patient's history and suspected condition, may jeopardize the quality of the care that the consultant can provide. Open communications among practitioners and between practitioners and the patient can help maintain the proper collegial relationships that benefit the patient.

At times, patients may be hesitant to see another practitioner, especially if they are concerned about the confidentiality of information that they have provided to the original optometrist. As expressed in the AOA Code of Ethics, respect for patient confidentiality requires that the optometrist obtain the patient's permission before disclosing the patient's information to other practitioners, and patients may legitimately request that certain information be withheld from the consultant. In 1995 the AOA House of Delegates further resolved through Resolution 1914 "that doctors of optometry transmit to other professional practitioners, upon written authorization by the patient, all appropriate information as designated from the patient's record; and ...that doctors of optometry transmitting patient records to another professional practitioner inform the practitioner when portions of a patient's record are being omitted at the request and authorization of the patient."[2]

Referrals and requests for consultation should be specific enough to allow the new optometrist to understand what care the original optometrist expects, and provide an estimate of how long the diagnosis and/or treatment should take. In cases where a patient's condition is too complex for a general optometrist to address confidently, the patient may be referred permanently to a specialist. This intent should be made clear to both the patient and the specialist. Similarly, when the referring optometrist seeks only to address a limited or short-term problem, all parties should be aware that the patient is expected to return to the original practitioner within a specified period. The consultant should follow up with the original optometrist to provide full information on the patient's diagnosis and treatment, again with the patient's consent. Unless the patient's condition is more complex than originally suspected, the consultant should make a good faith effort to return the patient to the referring optometrist for future care.

When a consultant is successful in addressing a patient's needs where the referring optometrist was not, the patient may request to remain with the new optometrist for all future care, or refuse to return to the referring doctor. The patient's rationale may involve anything from concern about the first optometrist's skills to simply feeling "more comfortable" with the new doctor. Whatever the patient's explanation, however, accepting the patient long term after the original request for care has been fulfilled would betray the consultant's collegial relationship with the referring doctor. Unless the original optometrist agrees to the permanent transfer, it is more appropriate for the second optometrist to restrict care to the purposes of the referral. If the patient refuses to consider returning to the referring optometrist, the consultant may suggest one or more other practitioners from whom the patient may receive primary eye and vision care.

The referral process of some MCOs and the qualifications of available providers in a particular insurance plan may also bring ethical concerns. At times the optometrist may believe that the level of care needed by some patients is unavailable within their health care plan or so urgent as to require referral to a practitioner outside the managed care network. In such cases the patient must be so advised and encouraged to discuss the consequences of pursuing such options with their plan's representatives. In the best interest of the patient, the referring optometrist has an ethical obligation to make every effort to maintain continuity of care by assisting actively the referral process.

Practitioners must recognize how economic incentives from a number of sources may influence their referral patterns. Most state practice acts and insurance statutes include prohibitions against "fee splitting," in which specialists pay a fee to generalists who refer patients without providing any actual services to the patient. Payment for referrals is also prohibited in numerous federal statutes governing Medicare, Medicaid, and other federal and state programs. Originally these types of federal prohibitions had the unfortunate effect of denying Medicare payments to optometrists who referred patients for surgery, even when they provided the original diagnosis and follow-up care.

Currently, however, certain co-management arrangements have allowed primary care providers to bill separately for diagnostic and follow-up services rendered in conjunction with treatment provided by specialists. Providers must, however, be aware of federal and state laws that prohibit certain types of business practices and referral arrangements, such as the federal and state anti-kickback and referral statutes and the Stark referral prohibitions against making referrals to entities in which the practitioner has an investment interest.

Both managed care and fee-for-service systems may create economic motives for referral. Under fee-for-service billing, well-insured or wealthy patients may be referred for unnecessary specialty services, often under the guise of comprehensive diagnosis and preventive care. In contrast, capitated payment plans may serve as a disincentive for referral if the consultant's fee would be deducted from the original optometrist's basic payment. Practitioners may be tempted to refer patients with conditions that are expensive or time-consuming to treat, especially patients who are poorly insured or indigent. However, it is illegal discrimination to refuse to see a patient solely on the basis of his or her illness or disability if the practitioner is qualified to provide care.[7]

Some manufacturers may offer optometrists financial incentives to use

their devices or prescribe their products. Such a commitment to a manufacturer may lead to unnecessary intervention or preclude recommending a
superior option for a given patient's needs, even if it results in no direct
harm to patients. As spelled out in House of Delegates Resolution 1886,
adopted in 1991 and modified in 1995, "...the American Optometric
Association opposes any prescribing and/or dispensing of ophthalmic products based on the participation by the eye care provider in a manufacturer's
advertising and/or promotional program involving the prospect of personal
inducements to the eye care provider from manufacturers."[2] Ultimately,
while optometrists have a legitimate interest in maximizing their practice
income, decisions about referrals and recommendations for treatment must
"keep the visual welfare of the patient uppermost at all times."[1]

Collegial Responsibilities to Impaired Providers

Through their interaction with patients and colleagues, optometrists
may learn of other practitioners whose work with patients appears to fall
outside accepted standards of practice, or whose personal behavior or
health status appears to endanger patient safety. A competent optometrist
should be able to make judgments that are based upon the patients' best
interest and consistent with professional conduct as directed by the Code
of Ethics of the AOA. Whereas optometrists must recognize and respect
differences in professional opinion and practice styles, the profession's
duty to safeguard the health and welfare of the public includes the responsibility to recognize and address behavior or circumstances that compromise practitioners' ability to make sound professional judgments within a
safe patient care environment.

There are many conditions that can impair the optometrist's ability to
provide quality care in a safe environment. Loss of professional competence due to physical limitations, failure to maintain knowledge, substance
abuse (including the misuse of alcohol and both licit and illicit drugs),
mental illness, communicable diseases such as tuberculosis or even the
common cold, criminal convictions for crimes against other persons, and
unprofessional conduct may all affect the optometrist's abilities. The point
at which a condition becomes an impairment may be difficult to establish,

but when patient welfare is threatened or patients are harmed by an optometrist's behavior or health condition, professional colleagues have a responsibility to address the situation directly.

Regulatory standards are intended to promote a safe environment for patients or reduce risks of improper practice. Continuing education requirements for license renewal seek to ensure that active practitioners remain current in their knowledge of essentials of optometry. State boards may suspend the privileges of optometrists who cannot demonstrate their participation in continuing education activities. Similarly, state boards may suspend or revoke the license of an optometrist found guilty of certain crimes, especially when patient safety may be at risk. Felony crimes against persons — particularly physical and sexual assault of patients, criminal possession of illegal drugs, and driving under the influence of drugs or alcohol — may result in the suspension or loss of an optometrist's license, in addition to any sentence from the courts.

Physical limitations and health conditions that could be considered impairments are often more difficult to identify and address. Aging optometrists may be at greater risk for physical impairments that can affect their ability to function professionally, as well as cognitive impairments that may affect their professional judgment. In many cases, the optometrist will recognize when physical limitations cannot be adequately managed and will limit his or her practice activities, work cooperatively with other practitioners, or withdraw from practice. To ensure that optometrists identify their potential physical limitations, take appropriate steps to provide a healthy environment for patients and staff, and safeguard them from the transmission of communicable diseases, House of Delegates Resolution 1893, adopted in 1992 and modified in 1995, recommends physical examinations for optometrists and their staff, as well as annual testing for tuberculosis.[2] It is illegal discrimination to consider age or disability alone in employment decisions, and employees with disabling illnesses have a right to reasonable accommodation in the workplace. Nonetheless, ethical considerations of patient safety must have a place in the management of the practice. Whether optometrists and their staff should be tested for communicable diseases, and whether patients should be informed of a practitioner's illness, depends upon the risk that the condition poses to patients. These decisions are typically left to the optometrist's professional judgment.

Whether in group settings or in individual practice, optometrists may not observe each others' interaction with patients, and it is often difficult to know whether a colleague is practicing competently and within the standards of care. Patients' reports about other practitioners' manner, conduct, or skills may be the optometrist's primary source of information about colleagues' work. Patients' complaints about other optometrists should be taken seriously, as negative commentary about any practitioner is harmful to the entire profession. Nonetheless, patients may not truly understand what should take place in an examination, and their observations cannot be taken at face value.

The profession of optometry is obligated to society to provide eye and vision care for the community as a whole and, therefore, optometrists should be concerned about the professional behavior of colleagues toward their patients. Except in those cases where the complaint against a practitioner is a charge of egregious misconduct that is required by law to be reported, professional ethics would encourage the optometrist who learns about a colleague's questionable practice to attempt to talk with the other practitioner about it directly in a non-threatening, collegial manner.[8] Such conversation should give the optometrist whose behavior has been questioned an opportunity to provide new information or another interpretation of events, and ask for or be offered assistance. A simple phone call may clarify a patient's misunderstanding or point out an easily remedied problem. A colleague's inquiry can provide needed support for the integrity of the practitioner and the profession as a whole. Sound professional practice cannot be so independent that such collegial conversation should be considered inappropriate. The professional commitment to a supportive relationship with other optometrists also directs the charged optometrist to receive such communications with an assumption of good will and professional collegiality, and even with gratitude.[9]

One of the greatest obstacles to helping impaired providers is that many affected persons fail to recognize their limitations, or deny that such limitations impair their care of patients. Denial is particularly an issue with alcoholism and drug abuse. When an optometrist is convinced of another's drug or alcohol problem and that colleague denies the problem or refuses to get help, professional ethics and many state laws and regulations require that the optometrist report the impaired provider to the licensing board.[2‡]

The optometrist who has cause to believe a colleague is impaired has an ethical duty to protect the public and to help the practitioner. The primary goal in dealing with all impaired providers should be rehabilitation rather than punishment, and treatment is readily available for health care professionals with a drug or alcohol problem. Typically, an impaired practitioner's good faith effort at rehabilitation will forestall or prevent action against his or her license. During voluntary or enforced rehabilitation, collegial support is also essential. Colleagues' help may be needed to cover the impaired optometrist's practice until drug or alcohol treatment is complete.

As a profession, optometry depends on its members' collegial interaction to maintain high clinical and ethical standards. The autonomy of individual practitioners is possible only through the common authority and trustworthiness of the professional at large. Through consultation and referral, individual optometrists extend their own abilities to help patients, and reinforce the profession's knowledge base through collegial communication and consensus about standards of care. Optometrists' collective obligation to the integrity of the profession requires that they be ready to help any colleague who cannot meet the standards of care, as well as colleagues whose professional commitments are threatened by impairment. This view of collegial interdependence is what sustains both the individual practitioner and optometry as a profession, and permits optometrists to continue to serve the welfare of patients in the face of challenges from within and from outside of health care.

---

‡ In some states an optometrist may be subject to disciplinary action if he or she fails to report another optometrist who may be practicing in violation of the practice act or who may be practicing while impaired. An optometrist should check with the relevant state licensing board for specific requirements.

References

1. American Optometric Association. Code of Ethics. St. Louis, MO: AOA, 1944.
2. American Optometric Association. House of Delegates Resolutions and Substantive Motions (compiled). Judicial Council. St. Louis, MO: AOA, 1999.
3. Classé JG. *Legal aspects of optometry*. Boston: Butterworth, 1989.
4. Helling v. Carey, 519 P. 2d 981 (1974).
5. American Optometric Association. Optometric Clinical Practice Guidelines (compiled). St. Louis, MO: AOA.
6. American Diabetes Association. Standards of medical care for patients with diabetes mellitus. *Diabetes Care* 1996; 19 (Suppl. 1): 8-15.
7. Bragdon v. Abbott, 118 S.Ct. 2196 (1998).
8. Moreim E.H. Am I my brother's warden? *Hastings Center Rept* 1993; 23 (May/ June): 19-27.
9. Ozar DT, Sokol DJ. *Dental ethics at the chairside: professional principles and practical applications*. Washington, DC: Georgetown University Press; copyright, Mosby-Yearbook, Inc., 1994.

Chapter Six

Screening, Testing, and Community Optometry

Satya B. Verma, OD
Elizabeth Heitman, PhD

"Screening is a good practice-building activity," stated Dr. Luther to her third-year students in the Principles of Practice Management course. "If you want to bring in new patients, do some outreach. Offer some vision screenings in schools, churches, or senior centers. It's good community relations: it will get your name in the papers and it will create good will. In the long run, successful screenings will draw in new patients and generate new patient care dollars."

On the surface, vision screening seems to be a straightforward, beneficial service that helps people and generates good community relations for optometrists. However, screening raises a variety of questions that make promoting one's practice through screening a gray area of ethical concern. The importance of screening depends on assumptions about the value of diagnostic information, early intervention, and the possibility of prevention or treatment that may not be true in all cases. Moreover, the availability of predictive information for given patients may have consequences for confidentiality and discrimination in the workplace and for insurance coverage.

Screening is usually defined as the application of relatively simple and inexpensive test procedures to asymptomatic individuals in a given population in order to detect significant health disorders or their risk factors. The primary reason for implementing screening procedures is to offer early intervention that will either prevent the development of a particular disorder or ameliorate its consequences. A second and equally important objective of screening is to investigate the epidemiological characteristics of health disorders in order to gain more understanding of their etiology and mechanisms, and ultimately to provide better preventive and curative health care to the public.[1]

Screening and Testing

The term screening is used differently in different health services and thus can be misleading for practitioners and patients alike. As it is generally understood in the optometric community, vision screening means using a standardized battery of tests on asymptomatic persons, often free of charge, to identify individuals with vision disorders that are prevalent in the age group being screened. Typically screening identifies persons with previously undetected signs of or risk factors for the conditions of interest, for whom follow-up with a comprehensive eye and vision examination is indicated. Screening also identifies persons with no abnormal findings for whom such in-depth examination is not immediately necessary.

Whereas diagnostic testing is carried out in response to a patient's symptoms or complaints, screening is motivated by the individual's *potential* to have conditions that often affect the population of which he or she is a part. Unlike testing for cause, screening does not result in a definitive diagnosis and treatment plan. Instead, its findings suggest the existence of a problem for which additional diagnostic work should be done to define appropriate treatment. For example, a tonometer may provide information about intraocular pressure at the time of testing, but by itself tonometry is not diagnostic of glaucoma.

In optometry the term screening is often used to refer to large-scale events in which a group of individuals with common demographic characteristics, such as older adults in a senior center or children at an elementary school, are evaluated at little or no cost in a community setting away from the optometrist's office. Unlike diagnostic testing in response to a patient's complaint, some levels of vision screening may be conducted by lay persons who have received basic training in the screening procedures, rather than by the optometrist. Many governmental agencies and service organizations use lay people to offer vision screenings in the community. Some have argued that when lay people conduct screenings patients are less likely to misconstrue the screening to be a comprehensive eye and vision examination, although lay screeners may over refer for follow-up.

Patient information forms about vision screening generally have a disclaimer that states that tests are conducted for screening purposes only and that the evaluation does not replace a comprehensive eye examination. However, many patients still believe that passing means that they do not need a comprehensive eye examination. This perception creates another opportunity for confusion about the differences between screening and a comprehensive examination.

Although optometrists typically do not consider their regular office practice in this light, many aspects of the routine eye and vision examinations for healthy patients can also be considered a form of screening. In the periodic eye and vision examination, asymptomatic patients are evaluated for a variety of conditions for which they have no symptoms. The recommendation that everyone receive a periodic "routine" eye exam is based on the screening philosophy that primary prevention and the maintenance of good health require patients to evaluate their heath status regularly. The difference between such office-based examinations and community screening is that the tests performed in the office visit are more complex and more detailed, and allow for immediate, personalized diagnostic work if anything suspicious is detected. A screening test may provide a tentative diagnosis requiring follow-up, whereas a comprehensive examination will result in a definitive diagnosis and care plan.

Screening as Community Outreach and Education

Beyond identifying a need for follow-up, screening programs may also be an important tool for community health education. Screening may alert participants to risk factors and symptoms of significant health problems, which they can learn to identify in the event of later changes in their own eye or visual health. The program should also educate the participants about the meaning of their own screening results and any recommendations they should follow based on those results. Moreover, community screenings can provide an opportunity to educate the public about the benefits of regular comprehensive eye and vision examinations. In this way, as Dr. Luther described to her students in the case above, a community-based screening event may create awareness of optometry's benefits and bring new patients to the optometrist.

The practice of conducting community-based screening as a form of outreach has critics, however. Not only may screening be mistaken for a comprehensive eye and vision examination, optometrists who conduct screenings may be accused of offering free screenings solely to identify individuals whose follow-up diagnosis and treatment will generate patient-care income. Such criticism may be valid if the optometrist is not willing to accept all patients who warrant further diagnostic testing, irrespective of the suspected condition or the patient's ability to pay for care. Reliance on lay people to conduct screening is thought to help dispel the public impression that the optometrist has a financial interest in the outcome of the process.

In some settings, optometrists who conduct community screenings may provide a list of several eye and vision care practitioners to everyone screened, enabling patients to make their own choices about where to get follow-up care. Providing such a list may also be important when screening is conducted by lay people, and avoids the appearance that the screeners are working to generate patients for one particular optometrist. Unfortunately, in smaller communities where there are few eye and vision care practitioners available, it may be quite difficult to avoid this impression unless the optometrist is known to engage in other community service.

False-Positive and False-Negative Results

Regardless of the setting or who conducts the vision screening examination, the validity of tests is a major concern in vision screening. A successful screening should be reliable, valid, and consistent — it should accurately separate those people who have risk factors and undetected symptoms from those who do not, and it should do so irrespective of the number of people screened. Tests typically used in screening often have high sensitivity — they identify as positive anyone with markers associated with the condition. Highly sensitive tests have a high rate of false-positive results, in that they may give a positive result due to factors unrelated to the condition being screened for. If a screening test is not sufficiently sensitive, however, it may give false-negative results, suggesting that an individual is unaffected by a condition that he or she really has because it failed to identify certain signs or symptoms.

Screening programs typically use tests that are highly sensitive, and thus have a high false-positive rate, under the assumption that it is better to refer someone for follow-up as a precaution than to allow a problem to go undetected. Typically, the more serious and/or the more treatable the health condition, the more sensitive the screening test should be and the more acceptable a high false-positive rate may be to health care professionals. Nonetheless, false-positive test results can create unnecessary anxiety for patients, who may worry even after more specific follow-up testing concludes that they have no problem. Screening tests that result in too many false positives also lead to over-referral, which adds to the cost of care and may raise suspicions that the optometrist offers free screenings as a way to charge for unnecessary follow-up.

Highly specific tests that would avoid the practical and ethical complications of false-positive results are seldom used in screening because of their typically higher cost and because of their higher false-negative rates. Still, no test can guarantee the detection of all "abnormal" cases. Unfortunately, for some conditions, there may be no single highly sensitive test available. For example, visual acuity measures alone may not detect certain refractive errors, and significant numbers of asymptomatic individuals may be falsely reassured about their vision as the result of a screening that does not include other tests, such as retinoscopy.

Irrespective of the sensitivity of the tests used, other factors that may affect the results of screening must be recognized and controlled to maximize its effectiveness and value. Both false-positive and false-negative results may rise with inexperienced or poorly trained screeners, variable testing sites and environmental conditions, unreliable or inconsistent testing equipment, and most importantly, patients' understanding of their role in the screening. For example, a novice screener conducting vision screenings for a large number of grade school children in a dimly illuminated room is likely to fail more children than the screening criteria for that age group would predict. Similarly, a student or a screener who is not an optometrist may refer more patients for follow-up in borderline situations for fear of missing a potential sight-threatening condition or risk.

The Benefits and Harms of Diagnostic Information

Before using any test for screening, a proper evaluation of the potential benefit of accurate results and harm from false positives and false negatives should be made.[2] Because no test can be completely accurate or predictive, there is also controversy about whether screening should be done for conditions that have no known means of prevention or treatment. In such circumstances the value of predictive or diagnostic information and the effect of uncertainty depends on the attitude of the person screened. Some individuals prefer ignorance to bad news that they can do nothing about. For others, screening offers the possibility of careful monitoring and life planning, even if the condition screened for cannot be prevented or treated. Some ethicists and preventive health specialists have argued that screening should not even be offered unless the person tested can use the information to take positive action.[3]

One extremely difficult situation in this area is when screening reveals a need for follow-up that the person cannot afford. Many optometrists and patients believe that it is better to undergo screening with no follow-up than to receive no eye and vision care at all. However, a patient who knows that he or she may have a serious health problem but who does not have access to follow-up evaluation and treatment may suffer emotionally as well as physically from the lack of care. On the other hand, once an individual learns that a significant condition may exist, he or she may make additional efforts to find the resources to obtain follow-up care. Although health care providers can generally choose whom to serve in non-emergency situations,[4] identifying an individual's need for care through screening places some responsibility on the optometrist to ensure that follow-up is available. Before undertaking a screening program, optometrists must consider how they will provide necessary diagnosis and care for persons found to need follow-up but who do not have insurance coverage or the personal funds to cover the related costs.

Similarly, providing screening only to those groups or in those communities whose members are likely to be able to afford follow-up care denies the benefits of screening to the poor whose need for eye and vision care services may be much greater. Such a practice is discriminatory, and runs contrary to the ethical goals of community screening to reach out to and identify those who otherwise may not receive needed eye care. The American Optometric Association Code of Ethics holds that, regardless of financial status, no person shall lack for vision care. In larger communities where the number of indigent persons may be too great for one optometrist to serve alone, collaborative programs can ensure access to the benefits of screening for the poor while sharing the financial burden among several optometrists.

Confidentiality, Discrimination, and Conflict of Interest

Others beside the person screened may be interested in his or her health information. Ensuring the confidentiality of the results of screening brings some difficult ethical issues for consideration. Employers in particular may provide vision screening to their employees. Their motives for offering such screening may not be entirely altruistic, and employees may not trust that their health information will be protected. For example, a transportation agency that wanted to provide on-site vision screenings to its employees received an overwhelmingly negative response from its bus drivers and train engineers. These two groups expressed fear that the information gained through the screenings might be used against some employees. Only when the optometrists and the employer reassured employees of the confidentiality of individual results did participation in the program increase.

The value of confidentiality is so important to the public's trust of health care professionals that those who would consider breaching confidentiality carry the burden of proof of any need to do so. Two recognized exceptions to the professional commitment to protecting confidentiality are concern for the safety of other specific persons and concern for public welfare.[5] An increasing number of states now require eye care providers to report those individuals whose visual acuity falls below a level identified for safe driving. Practitioners in violation of these laws face fines and other penalties. However, the specific requirements for disclosure of confidential diagnostic information to employers out of concern for the safety of others are not clearly identified legally. The optometrist may be better served to counsel the patient to reveal such information to his or her employer personally than to breach confidentiality by going around the patient to do so.

Nonetheless, employers may have a legitimate need to verify their employees' visual acuity. Some may contract with optometrists to provide mandatory screenings that will figure in the hiring and assigning of employees for jobs that require accurate vision. Optometrists who contract with employers to provide screening take on obligations to the employer that may conflict with their professional duty to protect patients' confidentiality.[6] The optometrist may continue to serve the interests of patients, however, by ensuring that the tests used provide an appropriate measure of the visual abilities needed for specific jobs, and that employees screened know how information gained from the screening will be used and to whom it will be made available.

Because most health insurance coverage in the United States is provided by employers, employers may also want workers' screening results in order to project their health care costs. Although the optometrist may carefully protect patient information, such information in the reports relating to services paid for by an insurer or managed care organization may be available to representatives of those organizations as a condition of payment. Once the insurer has this information, employers may also gain access to it.

Because vision screenings may identify systemic disease as well as visual disorders, vision screening reports may reveal information about the patient's general health to employers and insurers. Under the Americans with Disabilities Act, it is illegal and discriminatory for employers to make hiring, assignment, or firing decisions based upon an individual's health status unless it is directly related to his or her ability to do the job in question.[7] The use of screening information in such decisions is even more likely to be discriminatory. Screening typically identifies asymptomatic individuals who have risk factors for and previously unidentified signs of disease, without providing clear diagnosis. Nonetheless, employers and insurers may assume that screening tests accurately predict an individual's likely health status, and may seek ways to fire, reassign, or avoid hiring individuals predicted to have highly expensive health conditions. Optometrists can reduce the potential misuse of screening data by providing in the report appropriate interpretation of the findings for the patient's ability to work.

Ethics in health care is becoming more complex and optometry's expanding scope of practice makes the ethical issues for optometrists more challenging. Vision screening is often the patient's first contact with optometry, and it is essential for optometrists to recognize the ethical issues associated with screening. As long as a clear distinction between a screening and a comprehensive professional examination can be maintained, properly conducted vision screenings can do tremendous good for the public when the visual welfare of the patient is kept uppermost at all times.

References

1. Fukai M, Matsumoto D, Neumaier R. *Screening principles, public health and community optometry*, 2nd ed. New York: Butterworth, 1990: 85-96.
2. Shickle D, Chadwick R. The ethics of screening: is screeningitis an incurable disease? *J Med Ethics* 1994, 20: 12-18.
3. Mant D, Fowler G. Mass screening: theory and ethics. *Brit Med J* 1990; 300: 916-918.
4. Anderson GR, Glesnes-Anderson VA. *Health care ethics*. Gaithersburg, MD: Aspen Publication, 1987: 3-10.
5. Jonsen AR, Siegler M, Winslade WJ. *Clinical ethics*, 3rd ed. New York: McGraw-Hill, Inc., 1992.
6. Kamenetzky SA. *Fundamentals of ophthalmic practice—ethics and economics*. New York: Gower Medical Publishing, 1992.
7. Americans with Disabilities Act, 42 U.S.C. 12101-12213; 29 C.F.R. 1630.1-1630.16.

Chapter Seven

Allocation of Resources and Relations with Third-Party Payers

Michael Larkin, OD

Dr. Allen is tired. He often works a full day seeing patients and then spends another two to four hours on administrative aspects of his practice. Faced with declining reimbursements and market forces, Dr. Allen fears that he may be forced to choose between spending the amount of time that he wants to devote to each patient and limiting his standard examination time in order to increase the number of patients that he can see each day. Seeing more patients improves his practice income, but he is concerned that doing so may reduce the quality of care expected by his patients. Dr. Allen would like to continue to provide quality care and maintain a sound economic base for his practice. Although working longer hours has allowed him to meet both goals, he is worried that his own health is beginning to suffer from the pace.

Providing quality eye and vision care and maintaining a successful practice is a constant exercise in clinical and business judgment. While the American Optometric Association's (AOA's) Optometric Clinical Practice Guidelines for eye and vision examinations[1] describe recommended procedures for quality care, every optometrist is individually responsible for determining how to apply the guidelines and standards for each patient and his or her practice as a whole. Every clinical encounter requires the optometrist to consider how to use available technology and staff to meet the patient's needs in a responsible, professional way. The growth of managed care has created additional practical and ethical issues related to the allocation of resources, some of which can affect both the welfare of patients and the financial stability of any optometric practice with a large managed care patient base.

An optometrist's office may be a small, one- or two-person operation, where the optometrist handles all the patient care and administrative functions, or a large clinic with multiple providers, technicians, and clerical staff whose responsibilities require various levels and types of training. In any clinical setting, the essential role of the optometrist is to evaluate the patient, make a diagnosis based on the patient's history and examination, and recommend and perform one or more interventions in response to the diagnosis. Each of these steps requires the optometrist's professional judgment to determine which technologies will be applied and which staff members will take the necessary steps to provide the patient with the best available care.

The optometrist is responsible for a constant stream of decisions regarding the allocation of the resources to the patients that he or she treats. Many allocation decisions are made in accordance with formal standards of care, set by law, regulations, judicial decisions, or various professional organizations. Others follow with unwritten standards that reflect what most providers of the same discipline do for similar patients under similar circumstances. Other allocation decisions are influenced by the patient's interest in, demand for, or refusal of certain interventions, as well as by his or her ability and willingness to pay for treatment. Still others may be influenced by utilization review systems of third-party payers, which define whether and how much the patient's insurance will pay for specific interventions.

Often the optometrist's most important allocation decision is how to divide his or her own time among many responsibilities. Where to spend professional time is a question that also defines many issues of resource use. Where technological advances or the assistance of trained staff makes it possible for the optometrist to work with more patients or concentrate on specific aspects of care, when and how to employ such staff and technology must be considered carefully.

Technology, Staffing, and the Optometrist's Role in Patient Care

Technological developments have led to instrumentation that can reduce the need for the optometrist to be immediately involved in every step of the patient's care. Examination almost always involves data collection, and technology is available that can collect some necessary examination data for the optometrist, increasing the number of patients who can be seen. Automated testing using autorefractors, automated visual fields equipment, or corneal topography, carried out by trained technicians, may free the optometrist for other testing procedures that only a licensed clinician can perform, such as ophthalmoscopy, slit-lamp examination, Goldmann tonometry, etc. Computerized patient history taking using standardized questionnaires may also free the optometrist from the time-consuming gathering of basic background information, leaving more time for personalized discussion of the patient's specific questions or problems. Trained staff can also make notes in the medical record while the optometrist performs the examination, reducing the need for record keeping by the optometrist (and often increasing the legibility of the medical record!).

The computerization of medical records is another recent advance that can free the optometrist from repetitious record keeping and chart review, improving the efficiency of patient care as well as its quality. Computerized records can be developed to include the AOA's Optometric Clinical Practice Guidelines, allowing the optometrist to compare a patient's examination with recommended procedures in relevant guidelines, and offering a reminder of any special tests suggested to meet them. Information about patients' insurance coverage and third-party coding, prescriptions — including information about patients' allergies to medication and potentially harmful drug interactions, and even educational materials can also be incorporated into the computerized medical record. Patient-specific, computer-generated educational materials save the optometrist time in explaining treatment and diagnostic information by providing a template for the discussion. These do not replace the important time when the doctor talks with the patient, but rather reinforce the conversation and instructions with a take-home version of the essential details, such as dosage of medication.

The use of staff and technology to assist in providing care that was once the sole duty of the optometrist requires the careful training and supervision of assistants in order to improve the efficiency of the practice without sacrificing the quality of care to patients. Some states specifically limit the activities of staff and technicians, but even when they are legally permitted to provide services, the individual optometrist is still responsible for the outcome of care given by his or her auxiliaries. The more clinical activities that non-optometrists take on, whether to permit the optometrist to attend to other, more challenging clinical problems or simply to increase the number of patients seen per day, the more the optometrist must have safeguards in place to ensure the quality of care provided to each patient.

Medical Necessity and Quality of Care

Traditionally, defining the standard of care and allocating the resources necessary to meet the standard for specific patients have been the prerogative of the health care professions and individual practitioners. As is discussed in more detail in Chapter 5, the optometric profession has both formal and unwritten standards of care that should serve as the basis for the optometrist's clinical judgments about individual patients' treatment. Procedures and interventions required for treatment to be consistent with the standard of care are said to be medically necessary. Withholding or failing to provide medically necessary testing or treatment is generally considered to be unethical, as well as potentially negligent. Quality of care is often improved when the optometrist goes beyond concern for basic medical necessity to a more comprehensive view of the patient's benefit. However, overtreatment, or unnecessary testing or follow-up that are not in the best interest of the patient, is also considered to be a cause of low quality of care.

With technology changing rapidly and new methods of treatment and drugs constantly being developed, formal standards of care and published clinical guidelines may occasionally become out of date. The optometrist has the responsibility of maintaining updated clinical knowledge, and where there is conflict between the optometrist's patient-specific professional judgment and general guidelines, professional judgment should determine care. However, when an optometrist chooses to deviate from formal standards of practice, he or she should have a clear understanding of the limits of the formal guideline and clearly document the rationale for the alternative treatment plan in the patient's record.

Since the 1970s, the health insurance industry and employers who pay for many Americans' health insurance have challenged the ultimate authority of professional standards of care and clinicians' professional judgment. Typically they have claimed that fee-for-service payment systems create incentives for clinicians to overutilize services in order to increase their own financial gain, and that professional standards of care encourage overtreatment.[2] Concern for the high costs of health care has led third-party payers to define medical necessity according to their own criteria. Insurers' definitions of medical necessity consider basic treatment of an "average" patient, and outline what interventions the insurer will pay for irrespective of the patient's particular needs or interests. The difference between clinicians' and insurers' definitions of medical necessity can lead to ethical conflict for the optometrist struggling to make sound allocation decisions.

Managed Care and Capitation

Since the 1980s, as traditional fee-for-service health insurance plans have given way to managed care plans, decisions about the type and amount of intervention that a patient will receive have been made on two levels. First, many managed care organizations (MCOs) offer various levels of coverage based on the cost-effectiveness of certain interventions across their entire insured population. Second, treatment decisions for a specific patient are relegated to the "manager" of the patient's case, a clinician who has contracted with the MCO to provide treatment to the plan's members. In a managed care contract, the optometrist typically agrees to provide care based on the plan's pre-defined treatment protocols designed for standard patients rather than solely on professional judgment of individual patients' ability to benefit from treatment.

Managed care contracts may vary with the MCO and the groups that the MCO insures. Typically MCOs offer the optometrist or other health care professional a contract that describes the extent of reimbursable care that the clinician can provide to insured patients. Such contracts presume that the optometrist will provide a pre-defined package of covered services to all patients for a set reimbursement, without regard to patients' individual needs. Before signing a managed care contract, it is the individual optometrist's professional responsibility to evaluate the details of the contract with concern for serving the best interests of the patients covered by the MCO.

Professional standards of care do not consider reimbursement levels, and when faced with a "limited scope" contract the optometrist must be willing to consider patients' welfare first and foremost rather than letting treatment be defined by the limits of coverage. The question that the optometrist should consider is not "what level of care do I provide based on reimbursement," but rather "how can I provide quality care within optometry's standards of care and clinical practice guidelines, given the reimbursement levels of the MCO contract?" If the provider has concerns about implied limits on care, these issues should be resolved prior to signing the contract.

Some managed care contracts pay the optometrist on a per-patient per-month or per-member per-month (PMPM) basis. Contracts that involve capitated (per "head") payment require the optometrist to assume financial risk for the patients' welfare, since the provider agrees to provide care for a set PMPM fee. Some patients require more care, others less; the contract pays the same for everyone, whatever their need or use of services. Under such contracts the provider usually cannot charge additional fees for extended or complex care, leaving him or her at risk of not being reimbursed for services provided to patients whose need is greater than coverage limits. Such contracts can create incentives for undertreating patients, especially those with special needs, because the optometrist's income from such patients is limited to unspent funds from the prepaid PMPM fee.[2] In some cases, PMPM fees can be negotiated prior to signing the contract. However, once the optometrist signs the managed care contract, appropriate care is expected and always in the best interest of the patient. Reimbursement should be a secondary issue.

Capitated payment plans can also create incentives for optometrists to increase the number of patients in the practice and the volume of patients seen per day. Increased volume may compensate for reduction in per-patient reimbursement and allow the practice to survive financially despite fixed overhead and increasing costs. However, as illustrated by Dr. Allen in the case above, increasing patient volume also increases the physical and mental workload of both the optometrist and the staff. At some point, the increased volume may affect the quality of care by reducing the services provided, or by leading to provider exhaustion or other factors that may be detrimental to patients.

While there is no magic number of patients per hour or per day that can be seen in an optometrist's office, there are several indications of when a likely maximum has been reached. Before increasing his or her patient population significantly, the optometrist should consider a number of questions:

- Can I continue to provide quality care if I increase my patient load?

- Have I reached the limit of my own mental or physical capacity, increasing the risk that I might make errors in diagnosis or treatment?

- Am I so busy that I rush my examination and occasionally leave out certain tests?

- Do I spend less time with some patients just so I can keep up with the appointment schedule?

- Am I becoming unhappy with myself, my patients, or my profession because I feel overworked or burned out?

A "yes" answer to any of these questions suggests that the optometrist may have reached his or her personal workload limit. Reviewing patient flow and the office layout may facilitate better patient care and reduce work-related stress. Similarly, addressing the efficiency of the physical plant and utilization of staff and equipment may solve some of the concerns about workload. However, it may be time to consider seeking additional professional and staff assistance.

Utilization Review and Denial of Coverage

Another important feature of managed care that has had a significant impact on optometrist's allocation decisions is utilization review. Both

MCOs and many other third-party payers now require the optometrist or the patient to obtain prior authorization for even routine diagnostic and treatment plans. Such approval is almost always required for referral to specialists. Whenever the optometrist must seek authorization for treatment, he or she should carefully document the patient's condition and proposed care plan in order to facilitate a prompt approval. Clear documentation and explanation are especially important for authorization of treatment of conditions beyond routine eye and vision care, and the optometrist may need to discuss the need for care with the patient's primary care physician as well as the MCO's utilization review personnel.

Most MCOs and other insurance plans usually require their contracted providers to make provisions for emergency care, including having emergency contact numbers and "on call" systems. It is essential for patients to understand the options and procedures for emergency treatment and relevant coverage prior to seeking care. In the event that the contracted optometrist cannot render emergency services to the patient, a referral to a provider who can render timely care is important. If the managed care plan offers emergency services only through another provider, patients should be informed of the procedure to seek care and how services are covered. Naturally, the optometrist and patient may elect to treat the emergency condition immediately and deal with insurance issues later, but in such circumstances they should make no assumptions about coverage.

In some cases, the managed care plan may deny coverage for referrals or special services that the optometrist believes to be warranted. In that event, the provider best protects the patient by discussing the indications for the denied intervention, and recommending that the patient seek the care at his or her own expense. Patients have the right to know their diagnosis and treatment options regardless of reimbursement issues. If the patient has a cataract and the optometrist concludes that surgery will help improve the patient's vision, the optometrist should discuss this option with the patient, even if the managed care plan refuses to pay for the surgery. When the need for treatment is urgent, as in the case of a central corneal ulcer, the optometrist should discuss with the patient the need for specialty care and the potential consequences, including rapid loss of vision, if care is not provided in an expedient manner. The patient may then decide what course to take.

With health insurance companies' plans offering many options, many patients and providers can become confused about the real extent of coverage provided under specific plans. Patients often assume that their coverage is "all inclusive" and are surprised to learn that there are deductibles or extra fees for services and/or materials. Unfortunately, many patients find out about the limits of their coverage only when the insurer refuses to authorize needed services. Optometrists need to be prepared to counsel and work with their patients on several issues to help them understand their coverage and the optometrist's legitimate billing practices. These include: the utilization review process and the need for authorization for services and materials; how to submit claims in a timely manner; how to identify covered services and respond to inappropriate denials of coverage; and how to select potential specialists and facilitate communication between the primary care provider and specialist.

With managed care comes an increase in paperwork for the provider as well as the patient. Optometrists whose patients are enrolled in a variety of insurance plans or who themselves have contracts with various MCOs are well served to have one or more employees specifically responsible for keeping current with the provisions of major insurance plans and handling paperwork for utilization review and reimbursement. When the care plan and options outlined by the optometrist are not what the patient expects to be covered, the optometrist or an appropriate staff member provider should encourage the patient to seek clarification from the insurer. When the optometrist recommends non-covered services, it is often useful to outline in writing the care plan and the nature and costs of services and/or materials for the patient to review.

The denial of coverage occasionally leaves an otherwise financially stable patient unable to pay for needed services, or medically indigent. During the course of clinical practice, almost every optometrist encounters patients — both insured and uninsured — who require treatment beyond what they can afford, and all optometrists should have a plan for providing uncompensated care to their patients of record. As discussed in depth in Chapter 12, the optometrist must consider the uncompensated allocation of resources in light of the ethical principle of "do no harm," which underlies the professional standard of care.

When contractual limits on coverage or lack of coverage altogether affect a patient's ability to pay for needed care, optometrists have several options. They can:

- Continue to provide necessary care, setting up a payment system that will allow the patient to pay the bill over time.

- Refer the patient to a local teaching clinic or hospital where services can be provided at a reduced cost.

- Contact relevant charitable organizations, such as the Lions Clubs International, for assistance.

- Seek support from pharmaceutical companies, many of which have special programs to help patients who cannot pay for their needed medications. Optometrists should resist offering multiple samples to indigent patients. Patients who receive multiple samples may not try to fill their prescriptions and may cease treatment when the samples are depleted.

- If the patient is eligible, consider a referral to the VISION USA program, optometry's national charity for low-income, working families without vision care insurance coverage.

In addition to these efforts, the optometrist can continue to negotiate with the patient's insurer, and attempt to educate the relevant primary care providers, case managers, or utilization review personnel about the patient's need for comprehensive eye and vision services. Providing the best care sometimes necessitates becoming an advocate for the patient with other organizations and sources of assistance.

Auditing and Other Contract Issues

In addition to requiring authorization at the time that services are offered, most MCOs review the treatment provided to their insured population by auditing their clinical charts with respect to the quality and quantity of care. An important part of these audits is the review of providers' utilization patterns, and most MCOs provide utilization "report cards" for their providers. MCOs compare the provider's level and amount of services to contractual requirements as well as criteria for medical necessity. Often MCOs' medical directors determine whether to extend, modify, or cancel individual providers' contracts based on the results of such chart audits. These reports can help optometrists determine whether they are consistent with professional standards of care and whether they deliver cost-effective treatment. They can also identify whether and where the MCO's contractual requirements conflict with optometrists' ethical responsibilities to put the best interests of their patients' foremost.

Some MCOs and other third-party payers may intentionally or unintentionally discriminate against certain classes of providers. For example, some managed care plans cover services rendered by only one group even though other practitioners are qualified to provide the same care. In some situations such practices may constitute discrimination that violates state or federal laws. However, some managed care plans based on the federal Employee Retirement Income Security Act of 1974 (ERISA), which preempts certain state laws, have refused to cover services provided by optometrists.[3]

When an MCO or other insurer refuses to cover treatment legally provided by an optometrist, the individual provider should first ascertain whether the plan is one of the 60% nationwide that are ERISA based. Then the optometrist should contact the insurer to ask why the plan will not pay for the care in question. The AOA's publication *Demystifying ERISA and Self-Funded Insurance Plans* provides more information about ERISA plans and providers' rights under this law.[4] Whether or not the plan is based on ERISA, the optometrist should discuss the problem with representatives of the state optometric association, who may have more insight into the situation. In some cases, there is little a provider can do about discrimination, but in other instances, knowing the facts about these ERISA-based plans can be helpful in getting reimbursement.

For the foreseeable future, third-party payers and managed care will continue to be an essential part of the U.S. health care system. Optometrists will need to know how to work with insurers to provide quality eye and vision care to their patients. Optometry's ethical commitment to professional standards of care supports tailoring services to each patient's individual need. Nonetheless, insurers' concern for the cost of care raises legitimate questions about how best to serve patients' interests, and optometrists must be attentive to the costs of their treatment plans and allocation decisions. In the end, the optometrist should consciously place patients' need for quality eye and vision care foremost, and constantly work toward achieving this ideal despite constraints presented by the patient or third-party payers, and the limited availability of technology and personnel.

References

1. American Optometric Association. Optometric Clinical Practice Guidelines (compiled). St. Louis, MO: AOA.
2. Brock DW, Buchanan A. Ethical issues in for-profit health care. In: Gray BH, ed., *For-profit enterprise in health care.* Washington, DC: National Academy Press, 1986: 224-49.
3. Employee Retirement Income Security Act of 1974 (ERISA), 29 U.S.C. § 1144.
4. American Optometric Association. *Demystifying ERISA and self-funded insurance plans.* Alexandria, VA: AOA, 1991. (This booklet is available on the AOA member Website www.aoanet.org/members. Look on the Eye Care Benefits pulldown menu.)

Chapter Eight

Adopting New Equipment, Techniques, and Technology

Arthur H. Alexander, OD

Dr. Blair is considering adding a corneal mapping device to her office, as she wants her office to be as up to date as possible. She has learned through published reports that the instrument is helpful in the diagnosis and management of many different conditions, and that it should pay for itself through billing for provided services. Although she knows that corneal mapping can be useful in the diagnosis and treatment of keratoconus and in monitoring contact lens patients, she is not sure whether using this equipment in her new practice can be justified financially. She considers whether, in a few months, her new affiliation with a nearby refractive surgery center will increase the number of patients who might benefit from corneal topography and make the acquisition of the device more reasonable.

Optometrists are expected to keep up with the field's constantly advancing knowledge base and to keep their office equipment up to date. The obligation to stay current is a cornerstone of professionalism, and is clearly set out in the American Optometric Association's Code of Ethics and Standards of Conduct, and in The Optometric Oath. While scholarship is the foundation on which the practice of optometry is based, the application of that knowledge often requires training in new techniques and access to increasingly sophisticated and costly devices. Optometrists face constant pressure to outfit their offices and clinics with the newest diagnostic equipment, remedial devices, and therapeutic products, not all of which may ultimately prove to be as useful as they first appear. Optometrists' decisions whether and when to adopt new techniques and technologies and invest in new equipment raise important ethical questions of professional responsibility and patients' access to appropriate care. Moreover, the development of technologies surrounding testing and treatment based upon genetic information may soon introduce new ethical issues for optometry.

For many people the word *technology* implies highly sophisticated equipment or devices that require specialty training to use. However, health policy analysts and others interested in ethical issues related to the development and use of technology in health care use a much broader definition. The Office of Technology Assessment of the U.S. Congress has defined technology to include all devices, procedures, and drugs used in the provision of health care, as well as the organizational and support systems in which they are used.[1] This comprehensive view suggests that every aspect of optometry involves technology, not simply those that are dependent upon "high-tech" equipment. Nonetheless, the most significant ethical issues raised by the adoption of new technologies in optometric practice relate to "high-tech" devices, procedures, and knowledge.

Acquiring New Equipment and Devices

Judgments concerning whether and when to adopt a new technology are influenced by a number of factors. How patients within the existing practice will benefit from the new technology should be the optometrists' foremost consideration. Have the benefits and risks of the new technology been clearly established? Whatever the benefit, cost and patient convenience cannot be ignored, and the availability of the new technology elsewhere within the community is also an important factor. An optometrist who offers a service or product for which patients otherwise would have to travel great distances may provide a real benefit to the patient community and to colleagues. But careful assessment of a community's actual needs may prevent the optometrist from investing in a technology that may become outdated before its costs are recovered. Regardless of what details influence the final decision, there are a few guidelines that can help make the decision a sound one.

When considering the introduction of new instrumentation into a practice, it is essential that the optometrist become knowledgeable about the conditions that the device is purported to diagnose or treat. Sales brochures and advertisements often cite studies and expert opinion in support of their products, but these sources are more likely to meet the company's needs than the clinician's. Similarly, while sales representatives may be very well versed in the operation of specific devices, their limited understanding of optometry means that they may not be able to answer important, complex questions fully. Optometrists should examine sales literature carefully and investigate the fuller context of the device's development and use before making a decision to acquire it. At a minimum, it is essential to investigate the broader peer-reviewed professional literature and talk to colleagues who are familiar with the instrument and its use, particularly those who practice in academic settings where critical assessment is conducted.

The central question to consider in the acquisition of new instrumentation or implementation of new techniques is which patients it might help and how it might help them. Does the literature support using the new device for screening, diagnosis, treatment, or some combination of activities? A screening technique or device that will be used on most patients to rule out the possibility of a highly prevalent or extremely serious disease can be valuable for most offices. Techniques or devices that are designed for the diagnosis or treatment of a single condition may prove less useful in the total cost-effectiveness of the practice, because they would offer benefit to fewer patients. The more prevalent and/or sight-threatening the conditions that the technology can address, the higher the priority will be for having it in the office. For example, the Goldmann tonometer, although not a new technology, is a high-priority device for almost any office because it is used to screen for glaucoma. Finding this asymptomatic disease early is essential to instituting potentially sight-saving treatment, and the Goldmann tonometer is also considered a standard instrument to assist both in diagnosing glaucoma and monitoring the effects of its treatment.

The Cost of New Devices

The cost of any new instrumentation is also a factor in any decision to acquire it. Will there be a sufficient number of patients for whom the technology will be useful? Acquiring technology that is designed for the diagnosis and/or treatment of low-prevalence conditions may not always make economic sense. Patients whose conditions require an uncommon test or procedure can usually be referred to another provider for that purpose. However, other factors may increase the need to have such technology available. Some patients prefer to get all of their care from one provider, not only for convenience, but because they trust their own optometrist and his or her staff and are reluctant to go elsewhere. Moreover, if the new technology is not available within the community and patients must travel inconvenient distances to get needed services, it might be reasonable to add it to the practice with the understanding it probably will not pay for itself.

Even where there is demonstrated need for new diagnostic or therapeutic equipment, its purchase may create subtle pressures for the optometrist to overuse it. The need to pay for any new device may encourage its use for patients with only limited possibility of benefit, especially if insurance would cover the procedure. This is especially true in the case of screening and diagnostic technologies, where overuse may be rationalized by the "need" to rule out conditions for which the patient is at little real risk. Even without financial pressures, the mere availability of a technology often creates what has been called a "technological imperative" to use it.[2] Because there is typically no clear standard of care for the use of new technologies, optometrists may feel compelled to use a new device whenever there is an opportunity to do so. Many patients are similarly intrigued by new technologies, and may request interventions that they have heard about even when there is little reason for the optometrist to use them. Using any technology without a clear indication can raise the total cost of care, even if less discriminating use seems to solve the problem of the initial cost of the new device.

In the case of Dr. Blair above, the decision whether to invest in a corneal mapping device raises almost all of these issues. Dr. Blair's new practice may include several kerataconus patients, but she may not have enough volume of contact lens patients to justify purchasing a corneal topographer. She can probably refer patients whose eye and vision care would be enhanced by corneal mapping, although at some point she may have a large enough patient base to make such referrals inconvenient for the colleague who provides the test as well as for her patients. If she incorporates corneal mapping as part of her routine examination, she can generate extra income to help pay for the instrument, and she might justify the extra procedure as a form of screening, since she may find evidence of some rare corneal surface disease such as kerataconus in asymptomatic patients.

However, if Dr. Blair incorporates corneal topography into her routine examination, the overall cost of care would rise without a real increase in overall benefit to most patients. Although her patients might be impressed that she is keeping up with the latest technology, she may lose others who cannot afford the higher cost of a routine exam. By affiliating with the refractive surgery center, she may refer enough patients for surgery to justify the purchase based on a real need to diagnose and follow her patients pre- and post-operatively. Under those circumstances, the purchase would eliminate the need to refer outside her office for corneal mapping, improve patient convenience, and enhance her ability to give good follow-up care.

Finally, to ensure that corneal mapping is not used indiscriminately for patients with little likelihood of benefit, Dr. Blair should identify clear criteria for such testing, in advance of acquiring the topographer. These criteria should focus on identifying patients whose treatment plan will be changed by the information that topography provides. They should be consistent with the published literature on the use of corneal topography and re-evaluated periodically to ensure that she is neither overusing the device nor overlooking some patients who could be helped by testing. In the final analysis, the judgment whether to purchase or utilize this and other new technology should be based on how it will benefit patients and should never be based on an economic decision that may exploit patients or third-party payers.

Introduction of New Technology into Practice

Once the decision to adopt the new technology is made, it will become necessary for the optometrist to become skilled in its use. This process may be as simple as reading the manufacturer's instructions or it may require taking continuing education courses. Optometrists who are already trained in the use of a new technology may be helpful in familiarizing their colleagues with its application. Generally, the more invasive the technology, the more formal and comprehensive the training should be. For example, more time and effort may be required of the optometrist who is incorporating co-management of refractive surgery into his or her practice than of the practitioner who simply wants to start prescribing a new antibiotic.

Manufacturers often have educational programs both to promote new products and to train purchasers in their use. Occasionally, sales representatives may offer to provide on-site training in hands-on patient care. In such situations, the salesperson knows more than the optometrist does about the device or product, but the optometrist is still fully responsible to the patient for what happens in the course of the visit. Before a sales representative is allowed to demonstrate a new product as part of an actual patient's examination, he or she must be introduced to the patient, who must consent to being part of the demonstration. The salesperson's role and the purpose of the instruction should be carefully explained, and the patient should be offered the option of a standard exam. Patients may be uncomfortable receiving care from a sales representative, even if he or she is only assisting the optometrist, and any patient's objections to being a teaching subject must be respected.

Even after the optometrist is proficient in the application of a new technology, its use in actual patient care is also subject to the requirements of informed consent. As with any technology used in examination or treatment, the optometrist must have the patient's permission to use the new device or product, and that permission is based on the information that the practitioner provides to the patient. The disclosure of both risks and benefits is one of the primary distinctions between professional advice and the sort of promotional information that might be received in a mercantile environment, particularly in respect to new products. The optometrist must explain the advantages and disadvantages of the new device or product in a way that allows the patient to grasp the optometrist's understanding of the scientific evidence that supports the decision to use the new technology to address the patient's needs. Claims of superior performance or outcomes must be backed up with clinical research, and other options must also be clearly conferred, especially those that may be less expensive or pose less risk.

Occasionally, a practitioner may be an investigator for an experimental technology or may have access to a device or product that is not yet approved for general clinical practice. The decision to test an experimental technology on patients should be based on scientific evidence that the new device or procedure is at least as good as and possibly better than what is currently available. Research on new technologies should follow a carefully designed study protocol that has been approved by an appropriate research review board.[3] Optometrists participating in research or product testing must recognize that, typically, once a patient is assigned to a particular intervention, related treatment is defined by the protocol, not his or her specific needs. Most research randomly assigns patients to either the technology under study or the standard of care, and one group, by definition, will receive the intervention that will be shown to be inferior. In contrast, the application of an unapproved device or product outside of a formal study requires strong evidence that its use is the patient's only option for benefit.

Obtaining the patient's informed consent is even more important with the use of experimental devices or techniques than it is with new, approved technology. The patient must understand the experimental status of the equipment or procedure, and must be free from undue pressure or influence to participate in the study. Inducements, financial or otherwise, are acceptable only if the patient understands that he or she is free to leave the study and receive conventional intervention at any time and without penalty. Financial incentives can be inappropriately coercive if they lead patients to participate in a project that they would otherwise avoid. The optometrist should make certain that monetary payment or other rewards given to patients for their participation compensate them fairly for their time and inconvenience, but do not induce them to undergo interventions that may not be in their best interests.

Once new products have been approved for general use, manufacturers may offer patient samples to introduce the items into the market place. Free samples help defray the patient's cost of trying a new product, and manufacturers provide samples in the hope that both optometrists and patients will be sufficiently impressed by the quality and/or effectiveness of the sample to prescribe or purchase the product in greater quantity. While there is nothing inherently wrong with this practice, the fact that the sample is free and convenient should not affect the optometrist's educated professional decision about what is the best product for the patient's needs. Then, in the process of informed consent, the patient and the optometrist should make the decision together as to which technology is the best choice for the patient, with the doctor serving as the patient's educator and advisor. If free samples of the chosen products are available, only then should they be offered.

The Genomics Revolution

An example of a new area of technology that will challenge practitioners' understanding of clinical ethics is the exponential growth of genetic knowledge. Of all the health-related technologies of this century, none has had the impact that is anticipated from this area of study. Optometrists, like other health care providers, must be prepared to address the scientific revolution taking place in genetic research and the ethical hazards that genetic technologies may create. Just as patients now request their optometrists' advice on such newer treatments as laser refractive surgery and cosmetic eyelid procedures, they may soon seek their optometrists' counsel on genetic testing for specific eye diseases or such cosmetic enhancements as genetic eye color modification. By considering the ethical issues that may be raised by genetic testing and treatment before their widespread introduction, optometrists may prevent problems for themselves and their patients, and make the best possible use of the technologies that have already begun to emerge from genetic research.

Although genetic research first took off almost 50 years ago, its real promise has been demonstrated in the 1990s with the advent of the Human Genome Project. The Human Genome Project is a monumental research endeavor sponsored by the U.S. Department of Energy and National Institutes of Health, aimed at sequencing all human genes and identifying their respective functions. Originally projected to be completed by 2005, the project is ahead of schedule and is expected to be completed by the year 2003.[4] The Human Genome Project is based on two major assumptions: first, that all diseases apart from trauma have a genetic component, and second, that every individual carries significant genetic flaws. As each human gene and its function are identified, the ability to diagnose genetic predisposition to specific diseases grows daily. Many ocular conditions may be linked to an individual's genetic make-up, both primary ocular diseases such as glaucoma and conditions that are secondary to systemic disease, such as retinopathy resulting from diabetes. Although genetic testing is not common now outside of specialty medical practices, genetic testing is noninvasive and could theoretically be used to screen and test for conditions that optometrists already diagnose using non-genetic means.

Many of the ethical concerns that optometrists currently face in traditional primary eye and vision care will also surround the diagnosis and delivery of care based upon genetic information. A well-grounded understanding of the application of informed consent and patient confidentiality, discussed in more detail in other chapters, will be of even greater importance in this new area of testing. Informed consent for genetic testing and the limits of the confidentiality of genetic information are already the focus of significant debate. Informed consent for genetic testing is complicated by the uncertain meaning of genetic information. Genetic testing can identify many of the mutated genes linked to late-onset disorders even before symptoms develop. In some cases genetic testing may provide patients an opportunity to prevent or forestall the development of a genetically linked disease or decrease its severity. In other cases, however, genetic testing for susceptibility genes may simply inform the patient and caregiver that the patient is at greater than average risk of developing a condition. Unfortunately, many of the conditions for which testing is already possible are not preventable or treatable at present.

Because genetic material is shared by family members, the traditional ethical commitment to patient confidentiality is challenged by genetic testing. Not unlike the privacy conflicts that occur in the treatment of patients with communicable diseases, genetic testing for conditions likely to affect the patient's family members creates controversy for the practitioner who must manage the conflict between the duty to maintain privacy for the individual and the duty to warn family members of their possible risk. Currently discussion of the meaning of a genetic test and evaluation of others' need to know the test's results are usually undertaken both prior to (pre-test) and after (post-test) genetic testing. Through such genetic counseling the practitioner and patient can determine together the value of testing for genetic conditions that cannot be prevented or treated, who will need to know the results of testing, and how testing may affect the patient's relationships with family, employers, insurers, etc.[5] As with all clinical information with profound implications, the availability of genetic information may have a significant psychological impact on individuals and their families, as well as serious practical consequences if confidentiality is not maintained.

Optometry will also need to establish standards for the use of genetic testing in diagnosis and screening. The entire population will be candidates for some form of genetic testing and, theoretically, screening for predisposition to a range of ocular disease could include prenatal screening or even pre-implantation screening of embryos for in vitro fertilization. The possibility of implementing genetic therapy or genetic enhancements, although further away than widespread genetic testing, will similarly require optometrists to identify the appropriate candidates for such intervention. Decisions made by patients and practitioners based on present-day genetic knowledge may affect future generations in unpredictable ways, and their potential consequences must be considered carefully. Individual professionals also will need to become aware of the possible ethical, legal, and social implications of having genetic information available to patients and others, before they incorporate genetic technologies into their own practices.

Optometrists' work will almost certainly become more directly affected by genetics in the near future. As always, the need to learn enough about the technology to provide careful and compassionate counseling to patients will be of utmost importance. As with any new scientific development, clinicians must guard against the overzealous claims of the promoters of new genetic technologies, and evaluate their usefulness based on sound information.

Optometry and related health care fields are in a constant state of transition as new discoveries are made every day. New knowledge translates into better patient care only when the health professionals charged with the responsibility of providing that care keep up to date. Optometrists must assess emerging therapies, pharmaceuticals, instruments and corrective devices with a critical eye, evaluating the validity of the science behind the new technology and considering how new developments relate to existing technology and society's needs. New technology applied by a knowledgeable professional who puts the patient's interest first will fulfill the promise of new discoveries in providing improved health and quality of life.

Acknowledgment: Sincere thanks to Charles M. Wormington, PhD, OD, FAAO of the Pennsylvania College of Optometry for his comments and suggestions on the section on genetics.

References

1. U.S. Congress, Office of Technology Assessment. *Strategies for medical technology assessment.* Washington, DC: U.S. Government Printing Office, 1982: 200-01.
2. Fuchs V. *Who shall live? Health, economics, and social choice.* New York: Basic Books, 1974.
3. U.S. Public Health Service, Division of Research Grants, Clinical investigations using human subjects, Memo PPO# 129, February 8, 1966, and Supplement, April 7, 1966.
4. Waldman M. Human Genome Project aims to finish "working draft" next year. *Nature* 1999; 398: 177.
5. Collins FS. Shattuck Lecture — Medical and societal consequences of the Human Genome Project. *New Engl J Med* 1999; 341: 28-37.

Part II

SPECIAL POPULATIONS AND SPECIAL ETHICAL PROBLEMS IN OPTOMETRIC PRACTICE

Chapter Nine

Children and Adolescents

Dawn C. Kaufman, OD
LeRoy Kaufman, OD

Jane is a fifteen-year-old high school freshman, who has been Dr. Whistler's patient since she first needed glasses at age 7. Jane visits Dr. Whistler's office with the complaint of contact lens discomfort, dryness, and reduced wearing time of several weeks' duration. As Dr. Whistler reviews her lens care regimen, physical health, and medications, Jane suddenly says, "Please don't tell my parents, but I am taking birth control pills. Could that be the cause of my eye problems?"

Working with children presents some distinctive ethical issues. One of the most important features of working with children is the involvement of an additional party – the child's parent(s) or guardian — in the decision-making process. The difficulties that such three-way interactions can create have necessitated legal standards for the treatment of children. Federal, state, and local governmental agencies have adopted rules and regulations that guide the interactions of children, their decision makers, caregivers, and the public. Much of how optometrists interact with children is tightly regulated, and failure to abide by these regulations can have serious personal and professional consequences.

A second distinctive feature of examining and treating children is the length of time over which the consequences of decisions will be felt. Good and bad judgment and the results of clinical decisions can be profoundly magnified over time. Jury awards in liability suits provide adequate emphasis to this point. On a related point, the optometrist's interaction with a child patient is often the foundation for that patient's later expectations of eye and vision care as an adult.

Yet another distinctive feature is that childhood spans almost two decades, from birth through late adolescence. There is great variability in the needs of children of different ages, both in terms of their eye and vision care needs and how their different levels of maturity are treated.

Consent, Assent, and Refusal of Treatment

U.S. society values both the principle of autonomy and the protection of the vulnerable, and health care providers have struggled with these concepts as they relate to the care of children. Children in a clinical setting have no legal autonomy in decision making involving either testing or needed treatment. As the minor child is not autonomous, he or she cannot consent to diagnosis or treatment, and it is necessary to seek the proxy consent of the child's parent(s) or guardian who have the legal authority to speak for the child. In the last decade, the ethical discussion of consent for children has been broadened to include the concept of *assent*, allowing the child a voice in his or her care.[1] Clinicians have been encouraged to provide age-appropriate information and education to their child patients about planned procedures and to elicit children's willingness to participate before proceeding. Small children may give assent without fully understanding the explanation or the consequences, although full disclosure of possible discomfort is necessary. Older children and teens will understand more completely, but their apprehension must be dispelled as well. The goal of seeking the child's assent and the adult decision maker's consent is for the examination and treatment procedures to be a coordinated effort of examiner, child, and parent(s) or guardian.[1]

When the optometrist, child, and adult decision maker all interpret the child's best interest in the same way, the decision-making process for examination and treatment is simple and straightforward. This is the situation in the vast majority of cases in optometric practice. However, dilemmas may arise when there is disagreement about what course to pursue. For example, if the child accepts a recommended course of action but the adult decision maker rejects it, resolution may be difficult. Should the optometrist open the discussion to others interested in the child's welfare, such as a teacher or member of the clergy, who might influence the decision maker? Conversely, if the adult decision maker agrees with the optometrist's recommended course of action and the child refuses, the optometrist must determine at what point he or she can, in good conscience, force the child to accept the plan or abandon the effort to influence the child in his or her own best interest.

One approach widely used to resolve conflicts of consent to treatment is to communicate carefully the options for action — including no action, listing them in order of their benefit to the patient, and to let the child and decision maker choose from among them. This method both gives the child and adult decision maker a meaningful opportunity to participate in the decision, and defines their options in terms that link intervention and expected outcome. Often even young children can participate in decision making structured in this way.

Special consideration must be given to physically or mentally handicapped children in decision making, whether their handicap involves speech, hearing, motor, or intellectual capability. These children have hopes and fears similar to those of their age mates. They, too, should be involved in decisions that affect them, and are entitled to the special considerations afforded other young patients. Investigation of the child's needs and limitations prior to the encounter will allow the practitioner to customize the examination and subsequent treatment and maximize the child's participation and results.

An area where consent is required for legal as well as ethical reasons, and where seeking the child's assent is particularly advantageous, involves procedures that cause physical changes in the patient. Failure to obtain a parent's or guardian's consent for such procedures could result in a court finding of battery. Pupil dilation and tonometry requiring corneal anesthesia are two examples. While there is no doubt that these procedures are presently the standard of care and that their benefits are well documented, it may be hard for the optometrist to insist on these procedures when an adult decision maker refuses them on behalf of a child patient. The standards and justification for dilation should be explained to the child's adult decision maker. If consent is denied, the optometrist should document the refusal completely in the patient's record.

In the last decade, a factor further complicating the decision-making process has been the growth of utilization review by third-party payers. In particular, managed care organizations' role in facilitating or limiting patients' access to treatment gives them effective veto power over patients' consent. It can be difficult for the optometrist to be an effective proponent for the child if coverage is denied. Nonetheless, the American Optometric Association (AOA) Code of Ethics and The Optometric Oath speak to the issue of making certain that no one in need is denied treatment, and a sense of justice should also call us to advocate for the patient's right to be treated fairly by third-party payers. Similarly, if the child or adult decision maker requests authorization for some questionable or unnecessary item, the optometrist should attempt to be fair with the payer as well as concerned about whether the desired intervention will actually serve the welfare of the child.

Being an advocate for children's visual health may also include asking adult patients about their children's eye and vision care. Without question, if an adult patient presents with an eye health history of genetic origin, then he or she should be informed of possible effects on other family members and advised to have them evaluated. For patients with more routine conditions, however, the question becomes more difficult. Improperly presented, even the most well-intentioned question about a patient's children can be misunderstood and perceived as prying or as an attempt to solicit new patients. An overzealous approach to family history taking also may be offensive to some patients. While, ideally, the goal is fostering proper eye care for children, such questions should be well prepared and presented, with the underlying motives for requesting the information made clear to the patient.

Privacy and Confidentiality

In working with children it is important that the optometrist gain their trust. This is accomplished, in part, by showing a genuine concern for the child, giving him or her our full attention, conveying that our relationship is special, and giving children a "voice" in their care. Part of such a caring relationship could involve the solicitation and discussion of information that the child would not want other, less trusted people to know. In an adult optometrist-patient relationship, concern for confidentiality is easy to accommodate. With children, the issues of privacy and confidentiality present an ethical challenge because at least one other person is typically involved — the child's parent or other adult decision maker.

Obviously there is considerable difference between dealing with matters of privacy and confidentiality involving young children and those involving older adolescents. Small children and pre-teens have little privacy, as their lives need to be largely ordered by an adult caregiver, and will often be examined with the adult present. Older adolescents, who often live as autonomous adults in our society, will frequently be examined without a parent or other adult present. Occasionally, as in the case of Dr. Whistler and 15-year-old Jane, information will come to light that will provoke ethical questions. While Jane's medication may be a primary cause for her contact lens problems, her use of the Pill implies sexual activity of which her parents may not be aware. In many states, adolescents are legally able to obtain contraceptives and related medical care without their parents' knowledge. The larger issue of the risk of sexually transmitted diseases, including HIV/AIDS, among sexually active teens should be a concern for all health care providers, but confronting teenage patients or their parents with your concerns may have varied results, depending on the relationship with the patient.

Office record-keeping is a crucial part of any patient's examination and treatment, and the confidentiality of children's records is important in the care of children and adolescents as well. While the optometrist owns the record itself, the patient has a right to the information in the record. If the patient is a child, the child's parent(s) or guardian may claim a right of access to the information on the child's care. Information that an adolescent patient has asked to be kept private may be revealed if the parent or other adult decision maker has access to the patient record.

Moreover, because many children receive optometric care under their parents' insurance plan or managed care contract, others, including the parent's employer, may have access to information about the child that is kept secret from the parent. Parents may also request that a child's record not be released to a third party, due to the impact that disclosed information may have on the family's future insurability or health insurance costs, or the parent's employability. The optometrist must carefully document permission to release information from a child's record, as well as requests not to release records.

It is important to know state and federal laws concerning disclosure of information that a patient or parent or guardian has asked to keep confidential. If it is unlawful for the optometrist to withhold the information, the responsible parties should be informed of the law's requirements, and relevant notation made in the child's record. The doctor may be at a distinct disadvantage if a knowledgeable, but fearful, parent withholds information or denies treatment to prevent damaging information from being entered into the examination record. Similarly, if an adolescent patient withholds sensitive health information for fear of disclosure, the child's care may be compromised, leading to otherwise preventable harm.

Adherence to Treatment Recommendations

Each successful patient encounter has as its core the importance and necessity of building a trustful, working relationship with the child and his or her parent(s) or guardian. From the first meeting, through the examination, the discussion of findings, and the deciding of a treatment regimen, this interaction results in a level of understanding about the desired outcomes. The degree of understanding and the strength of the relationship are most acutely realized in the area of adherence to the treatment plan. When the optometrist is perceived to be sincere, capable, and acting in the best interest of the visual welfare of the child, and when his or her recommendations fall within a standard framework of expectations, the child's adherence is often assured.

Eyewear for a child who cannot see the chalkboard in school or antibiotic treatment for an acute conjunctivitis are straightforward and well within the ability of the child and responsible adults to understand. More complex vision problems, such as poor performance in school due to anomalies in binocular vision, or the need to monitor eye health conditions secondary to systemic disease, may be more difficult to demonstrate to the child and adult decision makers. The child may not understand the need for lenses that improve visual efficiency but not visual acuity, and may be reticent about wearing them. The parent(s) or guardian of a child with a medical condition that affects the eyes or vision may not understand why more frequent re-examination is necessary to monitor visual changes, especially if the schedule exceeds the number of visits covered by third-party payers. Treatment regimens that require the active participation of both the child and his or her parent(s) or guardian are the most vulnerable to non-adherence. When more than one treatment option is possible, the optometrist should spell out the strengths, weaknesses, and impact on ultimate outcomes of each option. Through explanation and negotiation, a "comfort level" can often be reached that achieves the outcome desired by the optometrist, balanced with the effort, monetary considerations, and time the child and decision makers want to invest. The optometrist's role becomes one of identifying and assessing all of the issues, and constructing a plan that everyone can follow.

Overstating the severity of a child's condition or its consequences in order to encourage the support of the child, parent(s) or guardian, or third-party payer for a recommended treatment is a common temptation for many clinicians. A case can be made that it is in the child's interest for everyone to take his or her condition seriously, and that some overstatement will motivate everyone to accept the need for the treatment and adhere to recommended intervention. However, if such a presentation involves false information or intentionally misleads the patient, adult decision makers, or third-party payers in their decision to pursue treatment, overstating the case may involve legal issues of fraud and deception. Careful assessment and communication of risks and benefits of treatment are a priority. Exaggeration should be particularly avoided when the optometrist's financial interests are involved.

On occasion a child's comprehensive vision examination will reveal an ocular structural abnormality or systemic health problem that warrants further examination by another health care professional. A full disclosure of the findings should be made to the child's parent(s) or guardian, with or without the child present, as appropriate. In order to ensure that the child receives the needed evaluation and treatment in such instances, the optometrist must often assume the role of case manager, coordinating the choice of consulting professional, securing appointments, transferring reports, and counseling the patient and his or her parent(s) or guardian when the diagnosis and recommended treatment are known. The primary care optometrist must be mindful of the competence and special areas of expertise of the recommended consulting professionals, and not be swayed by personal relationships or biases. Securing the best care for the child and supporting the patient's adherence to consultants' recommendations are most important roles.

Experienced practitioners have all treated children who present for an examination with reduced visual acuity, often at all distances, that is miraculously cured with low plus or plano lenses. Whether the child is consciously malingering, or suffering from a deep-seated emotional problem, the prescription of remedial lenses for emotional problems has been a debated issue. While some physicians endorse the prescription of placebo medications,[2] optometry has been reticent to embrace placebo lenses to alleviate visual distress. The optometrist must base such decisions on the results of examinations designed to rule out physical or systemic causes, and after a candid discussion with the parents or guardians, design a course of action acceptable to the decision makers involved. Again, the welfare of the child is paramount, and if true benefit, physically or emotionally, can be derived from low plus lenses where no other solution can be found, and where good follow-up can be provided, it is acceptable to prescribe them.

More typically, from the time a vision problem is first diagnosed, the ultimate goal of most young people is to abandon eyeglasses altogether. By adolescence many children want to wear contact lenses. An emerging self-image, sports, and peer pressure all play a role in this transformation, which can occur at varied ages and maturity levels. Each practitioner will develop contact lens fitting protocols to help children and their parents or guardians decide if the time is appropriate for such a change. The child's maturity and ability to understand the care needed to maintain lens quality and eye health need to be assessed completely. A thorough examination and successful lens fitting can have harmful results for the patient if lens care regimens and adherence to a proper wearing schedule are abandoned. Due to the increased risk of corneal problems from the mishandling or misuse of extended wear lenses, the execution of formal consent documents is usually required. Because lens care techniques are so important to eye health, the optometrist and staff must be alert to young patients' misinterpretation of instructions due to the volume of information dispensed in this new experience.

Adherence must be monitored at future examinations for as long as the patient wears contact lenses. Cases of suspected or confirmed non-compliance should be fully documented and the patient reinstructed on proper care. While legal issues usually dictate the design of contact lens dispensing protocols, the larger issue of patient education in the role of personal eye health is most important. We should not instruct patients simply to protect ourselves legally, but to ensure that young patients will have a future of safe lens wear and good eye health.

Suspicion of Child Abuse or Neglect

At the 1993 annual congress of the AOA, the House of Delegates identified child abuse as a major national concern and noted that, as primary health care providers, optometrists are in a position to recognize signs and symptoms of abuse and neglect. The House of Delegates passed a resolution encouraging schools of optometry and continuing education programs to include education on issues relating to child abuse and the reporting of suspected cases according to the law.[3] The intent of this resolution was to provide optometrists with the knowledge necessary to address a number of difficult questions related to the reporting of child abuse or neglect. First, it is essential for the optometrist to stay current on the signs and symptoms of abuse and neglect, and to know how to document relevant observations and physical findings accurately in the patient's record. Optometrists must know their state's legal requirements for reporting, as well as who among the community's legal authorities is responsible for investigating reports of child abuse or neglect. Similarly, optometrists must provide their staff with sufficient guidance in this area that all employees know how to report their suspicions to the optometrist.

Because it can be difficult to draw a clear distinction between the reporting of suspected child abuse or neglect and the violation of patient confidentiality, it is important for the optometrist to report only verifiable physical signs and events, rather than speculating on the causes of specific findings. While in many cases it would be easy to let the heart and suspicions overwhelm prudent judgment and verifiable fact, the optometrist must proceed with great caution, keeping the welfare of the child uppermost in mind. A wrongful accusation could have devastating results, not only harming a family, but also effectively destroying any hope of a trusting relationship between the child, his or her parent(s) or guardian, and the optometrist.

Even more than the care of adults, the care of children in optometric practice demands primary concern for the welfare of the patient, since children are often unable to speak to their own best interests. This heightened responsibility entails particular challenges of communication and requires a dedication to shared decision making and the protection of confidentiality that is unique to this population. The scope of practice and the specific nature of optometry allow us to unlock doors of potential for young people, whose futures are shaped by good eye and visual health. The world benefits when we practice our profession to the highest level of our capability on behalf of children.

References

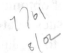

1. Bartholome WG. A new understanding of consent in pediatric practice: consent, parental permission and child assent. *Ped Annals* 1989; 18: 262-5.
2. Jonsen AR, Siegler M, Winslade WJ. *Clinical ethics: a practical approach to ethical decisions in clinical medicine*, 4th ed. New York: McGraw Hill, 1998: 69-71.
3. American Optometric Association. Resolution 1897, adopted 1993. In: House of Delegated Resolutions and Substantive Motions. Judicial Council. St. Louis, MO: American Optometric Association, August, 1999.

Chapter Ten

The Institutionalized Patient

Mark Swanson, OD

Dr. Faisal has been called by the administrator of a local residential care facility for the mentally impaired to evaluate Kevin, a 19-year-old profoundly mentally retarded man whom he has seen before. On previous visits Kevin has been combative and aggressive, and his previous exams have always had to be completed under sedation. He has been found to be a 3.00 diopter myope with 4 diopters of oblique astigmatism. Kevin has a history of self-inflicted injury including head banging. On two occasions, he has had to be pressure patched for self-mutilation of the cornea. The staff reports that he constantly bends his glasses, which are now broken. This is the third pair of spectacles that he has broken in less than a year. Each time the staff has been required to fill out an incident report. The administrator is concerned that he may injure himself with the glasses and asks Dr. Faisal whether he really has to have them. She remarks cynically that "the only time he really needs them is when the state inspector comes."

The institutionalized population constitutes some of the most vulnerable people in our society. The choice to treat or not treat, and determining how to provide the best care for specific patients within institutional rules, can be extremely difficult, as the optometrist may face conflicts between the needs of society and the institution and the best interest of the patient.

The institutionalized population, as we define it for this essay, covers a diverse group of patients in a variety of institutional settings and structures, including the military and Veterans Affairs facilities, long-term care facilities, facilities for the mentally ill and handicapped, and the prison system. In many cases institutionalized patients may have diminished mental or physical capacities that have led to their institutionalization. In others, patients may have no physical or mental limitations, but have constraints placed on their activities and abilities by the structure of the institution. Every institutional setting presents the optometrist with its own unique challenges, but there are some features that are common to all. While most of this discussion is directly related to provision of care within an institution, many of the ethical issues raised can also occur when institutionalized patients are seen within the optometrist's office.

The optometrist caring for institutionalized patients must often work within a system in which many of the rules and regulations are beyond his or her control and where the optometrist provides only one small part of their overall care. To ensure that patients receive the very best care possible, the optometrist must work well with a host of professional and nonprofessional personnel who may know little about eye care and optometry. The optometrist must work within the particular institution, not against it.

Basic Respect for Human Rights

Concern for "basic human rights" is often discussed in relation to abuses of power that occur outside the United States in settings unfamiliar to many Americans. However, the institutionalized population, by the very nature of their health problems and living conditions, present a special challenge to all who care for them in ensuring that their dignity and human rights are recognized and preserved. In The Optometric Oath, an optometrist swears to "provide professional care for those who seek my services, with concern, with compassion and with due regard for their human rights and dignity." The concept of basic human rights in health care has been expressed by many health care organizations in institutional bills of patient rights. These documents often state explicitly the group's or facility's goals in caring for their patients and the expectations that patients and families should have of those who provide care. These documents can offer optometrists an excellent framework from which to approach the ethical issues that they may encounter in delivering care in an institutional setting.

Consent in a Coercive Setting

In perhaps no other situation is the optometrist more in a position of authority than in an institutional setting. This authority comes not only from the natural fiduciary role of the optometrist but also the reality of institutional care. In many instances, a sole optometrist may provide all eye and vision care for a facility. While traditional ambulatory care allows patients to seek other services or a second opinion, this is often impossible for the patient in the institutional setting. In the institutional setting, the optometrist may need to work with patients who are unable to participate fully in decision making and who may not be able to give informed consent. These factors combine to make the institutional setting a potentially coercive or exploitative environment.

Coercion has several related definitions. To coerce may mean 1) to restrain or dominate by nullifying individual will; 2) to compel to an act or choice; and 3) to enforce or bring about by threat.[1] Coercion in each of these senses can occur in a variety of ways in the institutional setting. The optometrist may coerce patients into receiving an intervention that is not in their best interest, or that benefits the patient but produces disproportionate economic gain for the optometrist. The optometrist may compel patients to make particular choices by the omission of alternatives. Or the optometrist may need to use physical force or the threat of force to accomplish an intervention. The optometrist may similarly act coercively toward the institution, agreeing to visit the facility only when a set number of patients can be seen, or refusing to see emergency patients. However, the optometrist may also be the object of coercion by institutional staff or patients' family members who want the optometrist to intervene in a way that will serve their own needs but not help the patients. The institution itself may also try to influence the optometrist to act in an unethical manner in order to meet institutional goals.

As with all patients, institutionalized patients should be allowed and encouraged to participate in their health care decision making as much as is feasible, consistent with their own capacities and the institution's policies on patient rights and responsibilities. Institutionalized persons with diminished capacity are perhaps the most vulnerable patients within our society. They are often unable to provide any meaningful information about their wishes or even participate in the evaluation of their eye and vision care needs. Thus, the optometrist who evaluates them will have tremendous influence over treatment decisions. The severely mentally handicapped child with optic atrophy, the elderly person with Alzheimer's disease, the accident victim in a persistent vegetative state, and the war-injured veteran are but a few of these types of patients. Treatment decisions for these patients are frequently not clear cut.

The optometrist may be inclined to recommend a treatment, such as spectacles, that would be the standard of care for patients in the community, but which might be of questionable benefit to the institutionalized patient, especially if doing so would produce an economic gain for the optometrist. The Optometric Oath specifically addresses this issue when it states that "I will place the treatment of those who seek my care above personal gain." Nonetheless, as Dr. Faisal's predicament with Kevin in the case above illustrates, many factors must be considered in determining what is truly in the institutionalized patient's best interest. Whereas spectacle correction would clearly improve Kevin's vision, that benefit might be offset by the risk that he could harm himself with broken glasses.

Even where defining the patient's best interest is straightforward, the optometrist may coerce the patient into a specific choice by failing to divulge all treatment options. Doctors in long-term care settings may not recommend some procedures, such as cataract extraction, that would be beneficial to some of their patients, because of the difficulty in the logistics of having the procedure performed or limited financial benefit from undertaking it. The Optometric Oath calls for the optometrist to advise "fully and honestly of all which may serve to restore, maintain or enhance their vision and general health." However, even when the optometrist wishes to be faithful to this provision of the Oath, it can be a difficult task to provide full advice to the institutionalized patient with diminished capacity.

Many institutionalized patients have legal guardians or family members who serve as surrogate decision makers for all their health care needs. In 1991 the federal Patient Self-Determination Act mandated that hospitals, skilled nursing homes, home health agencies, hospices, and other in-patient facilities serving Medicare and Medicaid patients make known to patients individual state regulations governing consent to and refusal of treatment when the patient is incompetent, and the patient's right to make an advance directive.[2] Advance directives take two forms: the "living will," which relates to decision making in the event of terminal illness and incompetence, and the durable power of attorney for health care, in which an individual appoints a legal agent to make his or her health care decisions whenever he or she lacks the capacity to do so personally. While they are not universal, growing numbers of patients do have some form of advance directive that provides information on the individual's specific wishes about medical treatment at the end of life. Most, but not all, patients with advance directives want to refuse invasive, life-sustaining measures and accept only those treatments that will make them more comfortable. Unfortunately, living wills seldom address more general medical procedures, and while some eye and vision care may improve the quality of life of an incompetent terminally ill person, it remains the professional responsibility of the optometrist to determine whether such interventions would provide meaningful comfort during the patient's dying process.

Obtaining informed consent from a surrogate, whether a guardian or a family member or other individual appointed under a durable power of attorney for health care, typically requires discussing the patient's condition and options for treatment with that individual and helping him or her to come to a decision based on the patient's best interests. Again, while surrogate decision makers are likely to make rational decisions, they, too, may have difficulty evaluating the patient's benefit, and they may experience conflicts of interest themselves. At times the optometrist may face the coercive efforts of a surrogate decision maker whose wishes for a patient's care conflict with the optometrist's professional judgment about the patient's best interest. While families often have insight into the patient's status or preferences that should be explored, they may also fail to understand the limits of particular interventions for their loved one. In such cases, the optometrist must be prepared to work out a compromise or transfer the patient to another optometrist who is willing to carry out the surrogate's wishes or institutional demands.

Coercion can also become physical. Patients who are able to give their own consent do have the right to refuse examination procedures. In such cases the optometrist should warn the patient of the potential consequences of an incomplete evaluation and clearly document the patient's refusal. However, patients who are not competent to give consent may not refuse examination or treatment that their surrogate decision maker determines to be in their interest. The scenario of a screaming, flailing child who must be held for an examination is familiar to many parents. In such circumstances physical force is used with the parent's consent or often with their help. Similarly, the optometrist may have to use some physical force in restraining a patient who is apprehensive or in opening the eyelids of patients who do not understand or who are fearful of the examination. Because of the health and mental status of the institutionalized patient, the optometrist may be forced to coerce the patient into certain examination procedures, such as putting in drops for dilation, performing applanation or other forms of tonometry, and binocular indirect ophthalmoscopy.

The issue becomes less clear for the patient who is unable to provide his or her own consent and is resistant or combative. The line between what is necessary and reasonable force and what is abusive can be fine and somewhat indistinct. Generally the use of physical force to perform a procedure must always be considered in proportion to presumed benefit of the intervention. When there is a risk of physical injury to the patient or the optometrist, alternatives should be considered. Rescheduling the examination for a different day or performing the examination under sedation are possible solutions. Facilities may have standing procedures for examination under sedation with consent to such examination given at the time of admission. Except in the case of emergencies, if such consent has not been given as part of a standard admissions consent, the optometrist should seek consent from the patient's guardian before proceeding.

The optometrist may also become subject to the coercive efforts of the institution's staff or administration. Like family members, staff and administration may make demands of the optometrists that are intended to improve their own circumstances, rather than the patient's condition. For example, because the administrator in the case above was concerned about the paperwork associated with Kevin's repeatedly broken glasses, she appeared uninterested in any benefit he might get from improved visual acuity.

The optometrist must also resist efforts of the institution itself to have the optometrist act in a less than ethical manner, some of which may come, ironically, out of the need to meet multiple legal standards on a limited budget. For example, the cost of meeting an external requirement that all patients receive a yearly comprehensive examination may result in an institutional request that the optometrist simply screen patients. Likewise, some institutions may ask the optometrist to surrender professional optometric responsibilities to nonprofessionals whose services may cost less. Others may place limits on the services that the optometrist may provide, compromising The Optometric Oath's provision that the optometrist will practice to "the fullest scope of my competence." All of these are cases where the institution's goals and needs are not compatible with the high ethical standards of optometry, and where the optometrists must decide how to choose between them.

Lastly, the optometrist who cares for institutionalized patients must be able to distinguish issues of coercion from true oppression. Virtually all institutionalized patients may be coerced either by the optometrist or institutional staff to undergo or avoid a certain procedure or treatment. Such coercion may extend to the point where the patient has no real choice in some situations. It can be difficult, however, to determine when the coercion that is the norm for many institutions becomes oppressive.

The oppression of individual choice in order to serve the needs of the institution and its larger population can also be very clear cut. Within most institutional settings many personal liberties are already curtailed. Meals, activities, and sleep schedules are often highly regimented, primarily to serve the needs of the institution. A prison inmate who develops methicillin-resistant *Staphylococcus aureus* conjunctivitis may be forced into isolation and be required to undergo antibiotic therapy with no concern for informed consent. The facility's need to prevent an outbreak of this contagious and difficult to treat condition may supersede the patient's personal choice. More subtle coercion may become oppression when an institution needs to provide for the health and safety of many persons at the expense of one or more individual's personal liberty.

Substituting another's judgment for a patient's own choice is an enormous decision and should not be done lightly, even when institutional rules dictate. All possible other options should be explored before a patient's choice is overridden, and the patient's wishes and/or objections should be documented. Despite the constraints of institutionalization, the optometrist's primary duty is still to the patient. Careful planning and the exploration of possible scenarios with the institution's administration prior to their occurrence may make choices easier when the judgment of the patient must be overridden.

Privacy and Confidentiality

The Optometric Oath calls for the optometrist to "hold as privileged and inviolable all information entrusted to me in confidence by my patients." Protecting privacy and confidentiality is particularly difficult in the institutional setting. All patients in an institutional setting will lose some degree of personal privacy in both everyday life and in optometric care. The examination setting within institutions may be less than ideal. Examinations may take place in wards, personal living quarters, cafeterias, beauty salons, and hallways, where they may be observed by a host of others. Guards may be present during the examination of prisoners, and attendants may be needed for the examination of some disabled patients. Even in designated clinical areas within an institution, multiple patients may be brought to the examination area at one time.

In such situations ensuring patients' privacy is a major concern, both for obtaining accurate histories and for fostering the patient's trust in general. Whatever the institutional arrangements, the optometrist should do what is feasible to ensure patients' privacy. Some strategies include the use of privacy screens within wards or shared personal rooms, moving patients a discreet distance away from others being examined, and limiting nearby foot traffic. Conversation on sensitive issues, particularly during history taking and discussion of treatment, may need to be postponed until an appropriate venue is available.

A second area in which optometrists must respect their patients' privacy relates to the patient record. Unlike the records of most ambulatory patients in the community, the institutional medical record will contain a wealth of information about the patient generated by other caregivers, such as laboratory test results, which may be of significant potential benefit to the optometrist. This information can give the optometrist insight into the institutionalized patient not readily available otherwise. The institutional medical record will also likely contain sensitive information about the patient's social and family history. Optometrists should hold such information as privileged and inviolable as anything told to them directly by the patient. And because such information was gathered and recorded for use by caregivers unrelated to the patient's need for optometric care, it is perhaps even more deserving of optometrists' protection; since normally it would not be available to them, optometrists should even avoid discussing such personal and private information or issues with the patient.

The question of with whom the optometrist should share patient information is also an important one in institutional settings. By the very nature of most institutional care, the optometrist's orders will be carried out by others, and just as the optometrist has access to other caregivers' notes and observations, many others will read the patient's optometric chart. As Hippocrates stated more than two thousand years ago, getting the cooperation of others involved in the care of the patient is a professional duty.[3] The optometrist must balance the need to protect the patient's privacy with the need to ensure that others know enough to provide direct care that will serve the patient's needs.

Concern for the Optometrist's Safety

While the personal safety of the optometrist is occasionally an issue for practitioners serving a variety of populations in the community, it may be a significant concern for optometrists working with institutionalized patients. Personal safety must be considered in light of The Optometric Oath's provision that the optometrist will "strive to see that none shall lack for proper care," and with recognition that caring for institutionalized patients is almost always a matter of the optometrist's personal choice.

Threats to the optometrist's physical welfare may come from the risk of a patient transmitting an infectious disease, an accidental injury inflicted by a frightened, incompetent patient, or intentional violence. Optometrists who choose to work in institutional settings must be aware of these threats, and take appropriate measures to protect themselves, their staff, and their patients wherever possible.

Discussion of the issue of personal safety and the potential danger of working in an institutional setting typically evokes the image of physical violence against the optometrist. The risk of such danger is most acute within the prison system, where violence is a harsh reality. National statistics indicate that prison violence against staff is increasing.[4] While the optometrist is ethically bound to see that none shall lack for care, if there is an expectation for violence from one or more patients in a jail or prison clinic, such as a previous violent encounter, the personal safety of the optometrist takes precedence over the care of the potentially violent patient. However, the exclusion must be based on a reasonable expectation of violence from the patient and not simply an arbitrary concern. Just as measures can be taken to reduce the risk of spread of communicable disease, measures can be taken to reduce the risk of violence. Optometrists called to work in jail or prison settings must receive appropriate introduction to their patient population and training on the rules and procedures of the clinic prior to beginning work with inmates. Many prison facilities offer training to staff in how to avoid and defuse potentially volatile situations. Appropriate supervision of inmates during an examination is also essential.

The more common scenario for patient violence, however, is the unintentional harm that incompetent patients may inflict on caregivers out of fear or confusion. As discussed above, sedation may be essential for some procedures, for the safety of both the optometrist and the patient who may become violent in resisting treatment. As mentioned earlier, sedation and physical restraint should be used in keeping with broader concerns about the patient's welfare, and not simply for the ease of treatment of a recalcitrant patient who otherwise has the capacity for consent.

Historically, the most important threat to all health care providers has been that of the transmission of infectious disease. Patients with communicable diseases such as hepatitis, HIV/AIDS, tuberculosis, and methicillin-resistant *S. aureus* are common in institutional settings. Both The Optometric Oath and American Optometric Association Resolutions 1890 and 1916 call for the optometrist to participate in the care of patients with communicable disease and who are unable to protect themselves.[5,6] Notably, legal actions have been brought against health care practitioners who have refused to provide care to patients infected with HIV.

Moreover, the optometrist may be legally bound by the Americans with Disabilities Act (ADA) to provide care to individuals with chronic infectious conditions.[7] The term disability has been interpreted very broadly, and certainly covers many patients with physical and mental impairment seen in the institutional setting. The ADA severely limits the scope of cases in which patients with disabilities may be refused care and prohibits practitioners from refusing to treat classes of patients whose conditions lie within their professional expertise. The ADA states that services need not be provided only if the patient poses a direct threat to the health and safety of others. A direct threat has been defined as a significant risk that cannot be eliminated by the modification of policies, practices, or procedures or by the provision of auxiliary aides or devices. Fortunately for both optometrists and their patients, there are few infectious diseases that cannot be controlled. It remains the professional responsibility of optometrists working in institutional settings to coordinate with other affiliated health care professionals to establish and adopt policies and procedures that will reduce the risk of transmission of infectious diseases from institutionalized patients, and ensure access to as broad a range of health care services as possible.

Patients in institutional settings are often some of the most challenging seen by optometrists, and the provision of optometric care in long-term care facilities, prisons, and mental health facilities can be very difficult. Optometrists who provide care in these situations are to be praised. The ethical issues faced by practitioners in institutional settings often have no simple solutions, as the interests of the patient, the institution, and the optometrist may often conflict. As in the community setting, the optometrist should always keep the patient's interests uppermost in mind, but must also be prepared to do not only what is right for himself or herself, but to make the patient, attendants, and others cooperate in working toward the patient's benefit.

References

1. Merriam-Webster Collegiate Dictionary, 10th ed. Springfield, MA, 1998.
2. Patient Self-Determination Act, 42 U.S.C. 1395-1396a.
3. Hippocrates. Aphorisms. In: Chadwick J, Mann WN, trans., *Hippocratic writings*. London: Penguin Books, 1978: 206-36.
4. Bureau of Justice Statistics. Washington, DC: U.S. Department of Justice, 1988. ICPSR 8912.
5. American Optometric Association. Resolution 1890, adopted 1991. In: House of Delegates Resolutions and Substantive Motions. Judicial Council. St. Louis, MO: AOA, 1999.
6. American Optometric Association. Resolution 1916, adopted 1996. In: House of Delegates Resolutions and Substantive Motions. Judicial Council. St. Louis, MO: AOA, 1999.
7. Americans with Disabilities Act, 42 U.S.C. 12101-12213; 29 C.F.R. 1630.1-1630.16.

Chapter Eleven

The Elderly

N. Scott Gorman, OD

Mrs. Rosen is an 85-year-old widow who lives by herself in a suburban neighborhood. Her grown children live in another state. Mrs. Rosen is being treated by a geriatrician for mild hypertension. She tolerates her medications well and is otherwise in good health. However, she has suffered progressive vision loss and has been told by her optometrist, Dr. Soileau, that she has macular degeneration. Her visual acuity is 20/200 in her right eye and 20/70 in her left. One of Mrs. Rosen's friends, who is also a patient of Dr. Soileau, confides to him that Mrs. Rosen is still driving. She is concerned that it may not be a good idea, considering Mrs. Rosen's poor vision. At Mrs. Rosen's next visit, Dr. Soileau asks her about her driving. "Of course I'm still driving," she says. "How can you survive here without a car?" She is eager to point out that she has never been in an accident, only drives to the store now and then, drives "well below the speed limit," and would "certainly be able to see anyone crossing the road." She assures the doctor that there are no small children around and that she will be careful. Besides, she asserts, her side vision is "as good as ever."

The population is aging and the elderly, as a cohort, are increasing significantly in number. According to the U.S. Bureau of the Census, the 65 and older age group represented 12.5% of the population in 1990. This figure is expected to increase to 16.6% in 2020 and 20.7% in 2040. The fastest growing segment of the nation's population is the 85 and older age group. They will have increased from 1.2% of the population in 1990 to 4.6% in 2050.[1] These figures suggest that, now and in the future, senior citizens will be coming to optometrists to treat their acute and chronic eye diseases and vision disorders in greater numbers than ever before.

Increasing functional decline, dependence, and vulnerability frequently accompany the aging process. In a small portion of the elderly population, cognitive decline (i.e., dementia) is a confounding condition that places the patient at risk in today's health care environment. However, many elderly persons live in the community as competent individuals, capable of making informed decisions regarding their health care. Unfortunately our society and health care providers in general often do not recognize the capacity of the elderly. Respect for the self-determination of the older patient with capacity is vital for that individual and their relationships with caregivers.[2]

Many of the important changes in viewpoint related to health care ethics have taken place in regard to the care of geriatric patients. The importance of truthful communication and confidentiality has changed the approach to care of the elderly. However, there is still an inclination to treat an aging person paternalistically and to withhold the truth regarding his or her health condition. There is also a proclivity to violate the tenet of confidentiality by involving family members or significant others in discussions regarding the status of their loved one without the patient's expressed consent.[2]

During the 1990s, there has been expanding interest in questions of ethics in the profession of optometry. This interest has been stimulated by three broad trends: (1) advances in technology; (2) expansion of optometry's scope of practice; and (3) the increase in the numbers of dependent elderly whose care raises far-reaching questions of social and health policy. Although optometrists are not usually confronted with ethical problems related to life and death, there are many other important issues in the care of the geriatric patient that require thoughtful contemplation.

The At-Risk Elderly Driver

The case of Dr. Soileau and Mrs. Rosen illustrates a scenario not uncommon to the optometrist whose practice serves a large geriatric patient base. In both urban and suburban areas in the United States, especially in the Sunbelt region that extends across the southern portion of the country, elderly people want to maintain their driving privileges. Driving an automobile is not only an important form of transportation for them but is also a symbol of their independence.

National statistics indicate that there is a reason for concern when elderly people drive, since they have higher rates of fatal crashes per miles driven and per licensed driver than any other age cohort, excepting teenagers.[3] Elderly drivers do not respond well to complex traffic situations and, as a result, their involvement in multiple-vehicle accidents at intersections increases significantly with age. The rate at which traffic citations are issued to elderly drivers for failing to yield, turning improperly, and running stops signs and red lights is higher than that for younger drivers. There is also a higher rate of medical complications as well as an increased risk for death due to injury for elderly drivers involved in motor vehicle accidents.[3]

Optometrists have several options for counseling the at-risk elderly driver. They may advise the patient to curtail driving or cease driving altogether; to take a remedial driving course; to contact the Area Agency on Aging or other community resource for information on alternate transportation services; or even consider alternative living arrangements where driving would not be necessary.

Although most elderly patients will follow professional advice, some will not. It is this small group of patients that creates an ethical challenge for the optometrist. If the optometrist believes that a patient is no longer capable of driving safely, he or she has obligations to the patient as well as to the community. On one hand, as stated in the American Optometric Association (AOA) Code of Ethics, the optometrist has an obligation to the patient to maintain confidentiality and "to hold in professional confidence all information concerning a patient and to use such data only for the benefit of the patient." And as The Optometric Oath provides, the optometrist also has the responsibility to "hold as privileged and inviolable all information entrusted to me in confidence by my patients." On the other hand, the Oath contends that the optometrist has a responsibility to the community "to serve ... as a citizen as well as an optometrist." As a good citizen, the optometrist must not only do what's best for his or her patients but must also take into account the safety of the public.

A number of states have laws that require physicians and certain other health care professionals to report the names of persons whose health conditions may place them at risk for injuring themselves or others when operating a motor vehicle. It is not the intent of these laws to place the health care practitioner in a position to stop the patient from driving or to decide who should be permitted to drive. However, it is the practitioner's responsibility to alert the state's department of motor vehicles to persons who should be investigated based upon his or her professional judgment. To protect the relationship with such patients, the optometrists should inform patients that reporting is required by law, that their case is being reported, and that they will have a chance to demonstrate their ability to drive.[4] Whether and when to "blow the whistle" by reporting the patient to the state department of motor vehicles is a difficult decision to make. The optometrist's decision on how to proceed must recognize his or her moral obligation to both patient and society, together with an assessment of the relative risk of harm from breaching confidentiality versus the harm of maintaining it.[2]

The Abused Elder

Optometrists are increasingly aware that their responsibilities to patients and the community go beyond addressing the signs and symptoms of vision disorders and ocular disease. In the case of elderly patients, this responsibility extends to advocating for the rights of older persons to live a life of dignity and self-determination without threat to their physical, psychological, or financial well-being. When an elder's quality of life and safety are compromised, it is the responsibility of the optometrist to take definitive action, especially when the risk comes from physical abuse at the hands of others.

Elder abuse is defined as an "adverse act of omission or commission against an elderly person," [5] which may take many forms: physical mistreatment; verbal, emotional, or psychological abuse; material or financial abuse; passive and active neglect; abandonment; violation of civil rights; sexual abuse; and self-neglect. The common perception that older people are generally more vulnerable than younger ones is based on a pervasive and erroneous societal attitude that most elders are impaired and dependent. This notion leads to the elder person being viewed as having limited value to society and places him or her at risk for abuse. The presumed link between growing old and becoming dependent is in itself dangerous, and health care professionals should be committed to eliminating this ageist attitude.

However, elder abuse is a significant societal problem. It has been estimated that 10% of the U.S. population have been victims of elder abuse. Although elder abuse is a widely recognized problem, it is grossly underreported. It is estimated that only 1 out of 14 incidents of domestic elder abuse incidents (excluding the incidents of self-neglect) is reported to state or local governmental agencies.[6]

Although private citizens are not legally required to report cases of elder abuse, most states require that optometrists and other health care workers report suspected cases. Health care professionals involved in primary care are the individuals most likely to report and respond to elder abuse.[7] Specific laws for reporting elder abuse vary from state to state. In most states, however, reasonable cause to suspect elder abuse is adequate to support reporting, and definite proof of abuse is not required.[4] Optometrists can provide an invaluable service to their patients and the community by being vigilant in regard to the signs and symptoms of elder abuse. Practitioners need to become knowledgeable about elder abuse, aware of abuse indicators, and able to take appropriate action in a clinically and legally sound manner.

There are a variety of community resources that can assist the optometrist and an abused patient. If the practitioner suspects that the patient is endangered because of unsafe or hazardous living conditions, physical abuse, neglect, or exploitation, this suspicion should be reported to Adult Protective Services (APS). If the patient is a resident of a long-term care facility (i.e., nursing facility), the appropriate referral would be to the Long-Term Care Ombudsman Program, a federal program that was created to receive and investigate complaints by and on behalf of residents of nursing facilities and residential care facilities. However, if the practitioner believes that the abuse was assault, battery, domestic violence, theft, fraud, larceny, or neglect, the abuse may be classified as criminal conduct and should be reported to a law enforcement agency.[8]

Reporting of elder abuse involves the consideration of certain ethical principles. One of these principles is respect for autonomy, a basic tenet of ethics that holds that people should be free from interference from others. Second, the principle of confidentiality comes into consideration when information obtained during the course of a patient's visit to the optometrist's office results in a heightened index of suspicion for reporting elder abuse. If the optometrist reports either suspected or known elder abuse to APS or a law enforcement agency, the patient's confidentiality will be breached and autonomy may be undermined. Although removing an abused elder from a dangerous environment clearly serves his or her interests, reporting suspected abuse without the patient's knowledge or consent can create unforeseeable harm.

The Cognitively Impaired Patient

Dementia, a syndrome characterized by a significant deterioration of cognitive ability, results in a decrease in an individual's ability to carry out normal activities of daily living. It is a disorder that causes a decline in memory and intellectual skills, which may involve one or more of the following domains of function: language, perception, visuospatial function, calculation, and judgment.

Dementia affects between 3% and 11% of adults who are age 65 and older. The prevalence of this condition increases to between 20% and 50% in the 86 and older age group. The prevalence of dementia is reported to be almost 60% of those who are 100 years old and older.[9] Although many older persons who are in the early stages of dementia may live safely and comfortably in the community, decreasing cognitive ability and increasing age place them at risk for institutionalization. Whether a person lives in the community or in a long-term care facility, several ethical issues arise in the care of the cognitively impaired patient.

There is a tendency for the optometrist to become paternalistic in regard to older persons, and this inclination is greater for those who have developed dementia. Once the diagnosis of dementia has been made, patients are often classified as incompetent and denied autonomy, the right to self-determination. The optometrist should recognize that the clinical status of the patient with dementia is variable and many patients in the early stages of dementia can fully participate as partners in health care decision making. However, as dementia progresses, the patient's exercise of autonomy may need to be restricted, in keeping with his or her cognitive limits, but only in advanced cases of dementia should it be denied completely. It is important for all health care providers to treat their patients with respect and to help preserve their dignity, even when their cognitive abilities are impaired.

Confidentiality is again an issue that the optometrist must face in regard to patients with dementia. As long as the patient is able to make informed decisions and is not formally judged to be incompetent by a court, he or she retains the right to have all information concerning his or her health condition kept inviolate and confidential. As long as the patient appears to understand his or her eye condition, confidentiality should be maintained. However, patients with dementia may also make irrational decisions. If such a decision may result in the loss of sight or loss of life, it may be in the patient's best interest for the optometrist to breach confidentiality and to discuss the eye condition with a family member of the patient or other surrogate decision maker.

One of the newest additions to the vocabulary of clinical ethics is futility.[10] This concept may go back to the time of Hippocrates, who advised physicians "to refuse to treat those who are overmastered by their diseases, realizing that in such cases medicine is powerless."[11] Although the term futility customarily relates to the employment of extraordinary means for sustaining life, it does have application in the practice of optometry. Optometrists are sometimes confronted by situations in which the initiation, continuation, or recommendation of medical or surgical treatment would not be effective in increasing or maintaining the quality of life of a patient. For example, should the treatment of open angle glaucoma be continued in a patient who has had a massive stroke with a poor prognosis for recovery? Or, should surgery be recommended for a patient with advanced cataracts and end-stage Alzheimer disease? The new concept of futility in clinical ethics is a fertile ground for debate in the optometric care of cognitively impaired patients.

The Nursing Facility Resident

At the beginning of the 1990s, organized optometry began a concerted effort to bring to the attention of the profession, as well as to the public health community, the lack of adequate eye care for residents of long-term care facilities. This concern resulted from the recognition that there was "a serious problem...in long-term care facilities in regard to timely access for nursing facility residents to the services of eye care professionals."[12] Since that time, optometrists have significantly increased their involvement in the provision of onsite services to residents of these facilities. In providing services to nursing facility residents, optometrists regularly encounter two major ethical issues: the patients' variable capacity for consent and the protection of confidentiality.

Some health care providers, including optometrists, who work with nursing facility residents, believe that because an elderly person is living in a nursing facility he or she must be unable to make informed decisions regarding their care. However, many residents of these facilities maintain the capacity to make decisions even though their health condition may limit their ability to execute or act on their choices. It is important to recognize that the incapacity to make decisions is not always global but may be limited to "making a certain kind of decision or for undertaking a certain kind of action in reference to a particular time and circumstance."[13] For example, prior to admission to a nursing facility, some elderly have relied upon their close family members to assist them in making decisions regarding their health care. Subsequently, therefore, some residents may find it difficult to make a health-related decision because their family members are not available to offer counsel.

It is imperative that every attempt be made by the optometrist to respect the autonomy of the nursing facility resident. Not all residents of nursing facilities require skilled nursing care. Many simply have no other alternative, either because they lack family support or the financial means to live independently in the community. Subjecting nursing facility residents to diagnostic or therapeutic interventions designed to improve their well-being without considering their own wishes or desires should be avoided.

If a resident is truly unable to make an informed decision regarding care, a surrogate decision-maker should be sought out who has a clear and basic understanding of the resident's needs, desires, and preferences. This person may be a close friend or even a caregiver at the facility. In many cases such a decision maker may have been formally appointed as a legal guardian, or may be the agent named in the patient's durable power of attorney for health care. In most states, if no formal guardian or power of attorney exists, the law defines who among the individual's family is authorized to consent to health care procedures.

Maintaining confidentiality in the care of nursing facility residents is a second major issue that surfaces regularly at these institutions. Confidentiality is no less important to maintain in a nursing facility than in any other health care setting. However, because of the organizational structure of most nursing facilities, residents' confidentiality is breached routinely, even if not intentionally. Due to the close proximity of residents both to nursing stations and to each other, residents may overhear discussions among the professional and support staff, sometimes unavoidably. However, the optometrist should make every attempt to discuss the care of residents in a manner that does not identify who is being discussed.

The physical configuration of the area in which services are provided may also compromise the optometrist's ability to maintain confidentiality for residents. Most nursing facilities do not have traditional examination rooms, and services are often provided in large rooms that accommodate several residents at a time, such as the physical therapy room. Although this arrangement seems to allow for a more efficient flow of patients during the optometrist's visit to the nursing facility, it creates an environment in which confidentiality cannot be easily maintained. In such scenarios it is advisable to discuss a resident's condition with him or her either in a private area of the examination room or in the resident's own room.

The elderly population is a vulnerable one. The optometrist must be vigilant in his or her care of elderly patients, whatever the setting. Recognizing and advocating for the rights of the elderly to receive principled health care services will place the optometrist in a position to help to improve the quality of their care. Providing high-quality eye and vision care will, in turn, help the elderly to achieve their highest practicable functional capacity and secure for them a better quality of life.

Acknowledgment: Thanks to the Nova Southeastern University College of Optometry Graduating Class of 2000 for their inspiration and comments on the topics addressed in this chapter during their course in clinical gerontology.

References

1. U.S. Bureau of the Census. *Current population reports, special studies (P23-178RV). Sixty-five plus in America.* Boulder, CO: U.S. Bureau of the Census, 1993.
2. Ahronheim JC, Moreno J, Zuckerman C. *Ethics in clinical practice.* Boston, MA: Little, Brown and Co., Inc., 1994: 394.
3. California Department of Motor Vehicles and Beverly Foundation. *Teen and senior drivers.* Sacramento, CA: Department of Motor Vehicles, 1997. CAL-DMV-97-168.
4. Lo B. *Resolving ethical dilemmas: a guide for clinicians.* Baltimore, MD: Williams & Wilkins, 1995: 373.
5. Kosberg JI, Nahmiash D. Characteristics of victims and perpetrators and milieus of abuse and neglect. In: Baumhover LA, Beall SC, eds. *Abuse, neglect, and exploitation of older persons.* Baltimore, MD: Health Professions Press, 1996: 31-49.
6. National Center on Elder Abuse at the American Public Human Services Association and Westat, Inc. *The National Elder Abuse Incidence Study: final report.* Washington, DC: National Aging Information Center, 1998.
7. Baumhover LA, Bell SC. Introduction. In: Baumhover LA, Bell SC, eds. *Abuse, neglect, and exploitation of older persons.* Baltimore, MD: Health Professions Press, 1996: 1-5.
8. Nerenberg L, Haikalis SW. Discharge planning. In: Baumhover LA, Beall SC, eds. *Abuse, neglect, and exploitation of older persons.* Baltimore, MD: Health Professions Press, 1996: 207-20.
9. Mayo Foundation for Medical Education and Research. Dementia: evalu-

ation and diagnosis. World Wide Web: http://www.mayo.edu/geriatrics-rst/Dementia.I.html; accessed 12/29/98; last update 11/29/96.

10. Truog RD, Frader JE, Brett AS. The problem with futility. In: Monocle JF, Thomasma DC, eds. *Health care ethics*. Gaithersburg, MD: Aspen Publishers, Inc., 1998: 323-9.

11. Hippocrates. The Art. In: Reiser SJ, Dyck AJ, Curran WJ, eds. *Ethics in medicine: historical perspectives and contemporary concerns*. Cambridge, MA: MIT Press, 1977: 6-7.

12. Gorman NS. Optometric services in nursing facilities. In: Melore GG, ed. *Treating vision problems in the older adult*. St. Louis, MO: Mosby, 1997: 74-98.

13. Agich GJ. Respecting the autonomy of elders in nursing homes. In: Monagle JF, Thomasma DC, eds. *Health care ethics*. Gaithersburg, MD: Aspen Publishers, Inc., 1998: 200-11.

Chapter Twelve

The Indigent

Edwin C. Marshall, OD
R. Norman Bailey, OD

Mrs. Willis sat in the chair, withdrawn, confused, and openly apologetic for her apparent ignorance. Dr. Lorenz shook his head in disbelief. He hadn't planned on her coming in today. He presumed, like most health care providers in his area, that low-income people don't show up for scheduled appointments. He reminded himself that he had a paying patient waiting for him while he tried to explain a complicated diagnosis to this indigent, uneducated woman. "She probably won't comply with my treatment recommendations no matter what I say," he thought, "and she'll most likely try to sue me for malpractice when her vision gets worse." Although Dr. Lorenz was sitting next to her, Mrs. Willis felt alone and scared. She had never heard of glaucoma before, and the possibility of losing her sight was devastating and emotionally overpowering. However, she could tell by Dr. Lorenz's body language that she was keeping him from other duties, and she didn't want to waste any more of his time with her problems.

Clinicians frequently categorize their patients according to specific characteristics, especially when the characteristics have a potential for impacting clinical decision making. Epidemiological risk for certain diseases, the prevalence of certain clinical findings, and other categorical measures of clinical importance can be significant determinants of treatment that may warrant such labeling of individual patients. Some clinicians, however, may also categorize patients in terms of non-clinical factors, such as age, ethnicity, disability, source of payment, and related personal characteristics, including factors that may make the optometrist personally uncomfortable. At times such categorization may adversely affect clinical decision making and quality of care, as well as limit patients' access to professional services.

Economic factors, and in particular the patient's ability to pay for care, have begun to have a very strong influence on health care decision making and the delivery of health care services. Many health systems analysts contend that a growing number of patients find it difficult to achieve and maintain the financial support necessary to cover the costs of health care for themselves and their families. Increasingly optometrists are tempted to categorize by ability to pay, dividing their practice mentally into patients who can pay for all their care, those whose payment will be restricted by managed care contracts, and those who can pay little or nothing for the optometrist's services.

Because of various personal and social circumstances, sometimes beyond their control, large numbers of people in both urban and rural communities are unable to pay for health care. For some, the inability to afford health care is one component of a general inability to pay for food, clothing, and shelter: as a group such individuals are often called the *economically indigent.* Others may be able to meet their basic living expenses, but not the additional cost of health care: this group is increasingly known as the *medically indigent.* In either case, people who need health care but cannot afford it present formidable practical and ethical challenges to health care providers.

The Code of Ethics of the American Optometric Association (AOA) offers considerable guidance on the optometrist's responsibilities to indigent patients.[1] The Code calls for optometrists to see that no one lacks for optometric care because of limited financial resources. Moreover, regardless of the patient's ability to pay or source of payment for treatment, as professionals, optometrists are bound by a fiduciary responsibility to keep concern for their patients' welfare uppermost at all times. Embedded in the therapeutic relationship is also the assumption that optometrists will serve as advocates for their patients and their patients' health care. This advocacy is particularly important for indigent patients who often feel disenfranchised and lost within the bureaucratic maze of the country's health care delivery systems.

Professional Responsibilities and Quality of Care

Serving the indigent is a matter of both professional ethical responsibility and personal choice for optometrists. The Code of Ethics places great responsibility upon the practicing optometrist for the care of indigent patients. However, this does not mean that a practitioner is required, legally or ethically, to see every patient who shows up at the office, or to provide all the care that may be needed or expected by every patient. Health care professionals are not obliged to serve the needs of some patients to the point of neglecting their obligations to other patients and other professional responsibilities.[2]

Across the health professions, while individual practitioners are encouraged to provide care to all who seek it, there is no ethical or legal obligation for any caregiver to provide professional services to anyone outside of an established relationship, except in an emergency or when no other practitioner is available, as may occur in some isolated communities.[3] However, when a potential patient comes to the optometrist's office with a problem within the optometrist's expertise, the practitioner should ensure, at a minimum, that no additional harm will come to the patient if he or she refuses to provide treatment. In such cases, the ethical principle of *primum non nocere*—first do no harm—should dictate how the optometrist responds.

Once an optometrist decides to take on an indigent patient, he or she then faces the practical ethical question of how to define appropriate care for someone who cannot pay for treatment. The AOA's Clinical Practice Guidelines provide an important baseline for determining the appropriate level of care, irrespective of the patient's ability to pay. However, managed care contracts have institutionalized the distinction between optimal care and adequate care, which may appear to some optometrists to justify providing a reduced level of care rather than no care to patients who are economically or medically indigent.

The amount of time that practitioners spend with patients with different abilities to pay or sources of payment for care is also becoming more of an issue for optometrists. Under managed care contracts, many optometrists now must see significantly more patients to generate the same income that they did in a fee-for-service arrangement, and some may claim that the need to treat more patients demands shortening the time spent with each. As in the case of Dr. Lorenz and Mrs. Willis, indigent patients may be less well educated, and thus less knowledgeable about what level of health care to expect, than financially secure patients. They also may have lower expectations of potential health care outcomes. Nonetheless, optometrists must refrain from the socially unjust temptation to provide less care to the indigent than they would to those who are more informed or those with higher expectations.

The practice of providing a lesser level of treatment for the indigent is sometimes supported by the rationalization that, because a little care is better than nothing, providing less than optimal care without charge to the indigent is ethically preferable to providing no indigent care at all. The rationale continues with the argument that providing higher levels of care may actually reduce the number of indigent patients that the optometrist can serve, and that rationing services to a minimum acceptable level allows the benefit to be extended to a greater number of needy patients. The rationalization may be stretched further by a belief that indigent patients should appreciate whatever free care they receive, even if it falls below the standard used for paying patients.

Ever-increasing economic pressures may make it difficult for optometrists to assume additional financial loss either through reduced fees or nonpayment when they are asked to treat indigent patients. However, while providing eye and vision care for the indigent frequently requires the optometrist to make a financial sacrifice, economic considerations should not interfere with the primacy of the optometrist's commitment to his or her patients.[4] Health care providers operate under the social, professional, and ethical obligation to promote the welfare of their patients — whenever a practitioner fails to provide the best care because of financial considerations, he or she violates that obligation and compromises the professional responsibility of beneficence.[5] Once the optometrist accepts a person as a patient there is little professional discretion relative to the quality of care to be provided.[6]

Where quality of care raises ethical concerns in the provision of uncomplicated primary care for asymptomatic patients, follow-up and/or referral for indigent patients with chronic or advanced conditions can be extremely difficult. Unfortunately, discontinuity of care may be the norm for people without the financial means to seek and maintain adequate health care. If they are seen at all, it may be only once, sporadically, or by a different provider at each visit. In most cases, care is compromised by the lack of continuity with a familiar provider.

This difficulty is particularly evident in health screening. Without the intervention and assistance of concerned providers, follow-up or extended care may be inaccessible to indigent patients who have positive findings from a screening. Because screening may create awareness of a treatable problem but emphasize the patient's inability to get treatment, some critics contend that vision and eye health screenings for the poor may not be a benefit. Moreover, even where initial follow-up is possible, indigent patients' adherence to recommended treatment protocols is affected by their limited access to care, and optimal treatment is often compromised by the difficulty of monitoring adherence. Optometrists who work with indigent patients who change residences and move in and out of different provider service areas — especially seasonal or migrant workers and the homeless — may find it virtually impossible to initiate treatment programs and maintain continuity of care.

Patient Advocacy

Indigent patients, like all patients, entrust the health of their eyes to the optometrist who cares for them. Moreover, because of their financial need, indigent patients may look more frequently to their optometrist to represent their interests to outside parties. Often the optometrist can negotiate the supplementary support necessary to provide for the eye and vision care of indigent patients, making continuity of care more possible. At times the optometrist may be able to reserve office samples for their indigent patients, or work with suppliers to provide prescriptions and other extended services at a reduced or no charge. Samples, however, are also a limited resource, and dependence on their availability can complicate treatment plans. Advocacy with suppliers and other providers, too, may require too much time and effort to be feasible for many practitioners. Instead, the optometrist's assistance may have to be limited to helping needy patients identify governmental and charitable resources, or to making a direct appeal to local agencies or community organizations for assistance.

Governmental Programs for Optometric Care

Across the United States, eye and vision care are provided to some indigent patients through tax-based governmental programs such as Medicaid. In some cases, the poor may receive more adequate care through such programs than is available to the near poor and others who pay for eye and vision care themselves. In other cases, however, the benefits provided by a program may be insufficient to address all of the eye and vision problems that a beneficiary may experience. Under such circumstances the optometrist may regularly be forced to tell covered patients that their benefits under a particular program do not provide the treatment that is best for them. Then the optometrist is placed in the position of being an arbiter between the needs of the patient and the limits of the governmental program's coverage.

Because Medicaid reimburses optometrists at a level that may be lower than the actual costs of care, optometrists who treat a large number of Medicaid patients may feel that they are discharging their entire responsibility for indigent care without taking on non-paying patients. Other optometrists may not accept Medicaid, even if they do treat non-paying patients, because they consider the level of reimbursement to be inadequate and because the program's paperwork itself can be quite time-consuming.

The question of whether an optometrist may ethically refuse to participate in governmental entitlement programs because of their low level of reimbursement is shaped by the definition of professional responsibility. Where the professional practice of optometry is seen as a privilege derived from state licensure, the practitioner is thought to have public obligations unlike those placed upon the average individual in business.[7] By accepting society's franchise to care for the eye and visual welfare of the public, the optometrist takes on a professional responsibility to provide services to those in need, irrespective of their ability to pay or source of payment. Since the AOA Code of Ethics calls for the optometrist to see that no one lacks for visual care regardless of ability to pay,[8] the optometrist should not refuse to treat patients who are covered by Medicaid unless some other arrangement can be made to provide them with care.

From another perspective, health care has been likened to a social utility — similar to gas and electricity — in that it is a necessary service that people cannot forgo for very long periods of time. As such, it is incumbent upon society to make certain that the "health care utility" is universally available and accessible, and incumbent upon health care professionals to work toward the establishment of social mechanism that ensure this accessibility. Whether or not they favor Medicaid, optometrists have a responsibility as citizens and professionals to try to improve governmental programs that seek to provide care to the indigent.

Civic Organizations and Charity Care

Many individuals and families that qualify as indigent are not necessarily eligible for Medicaid or other governmental programs for the poor. The meager incomes of the "near poor" may exceed federal or state eligibility guidelines, even if they do not work a sufficient number of hours to participate in employment-based programs. For those who "fall through the cracks" between governmental and private insurance programs and who have insufficient income to fund their own health care, there are few options for comprehensive optometric services. The optometrist, instead, may need to rely on local charities to help provide adequate treatment for patients with demonstrated eye and vision care needs.

Most communities have non-governmental organizations that assist the indigent with eye and vision care, including such civic organizations as Lions Clubs International and Prevent Blindness America. The Lions have sight conservation as one of their major missions, and community branches of Prevent Blindness America often make arrangements with local eye care practitioners and opticians to provide care for individuals who fall outside the governmental safety net. Organizations supported by the United Way and other community-based groups routinely sponsor programs and activities to care for the specific needs of indigent and low-income groups. Religious organizations and individual congregations may also provide financial resources to underserved individuals and families.

Optometrists should be familiar with the resources available in their respective communities that help the indigent secure access to needed eye and vision care. As professionals and as citizens, optometrists should consider becoming active members in at least one such organization serving their community as well as taking part in projects organized by professional optometric groups aimed at improving the health of the indigent. Such activities may range from fund raising to serving at charity clinics that treat the poor. In addition, the contribution of leadership as a member of the policy-making board of a community-based organization can give tremendous support to health care for the indigent, and help to educate the community on the importance of good eye and vision health.

In 1985, the AOA identified the need for a national program of charitable service for uninsured, low-income workers and their families who have no other means of obtaining basic eye and vision care services.[9] The Volunteers In Service In Our Nation (VISION) USA program started as a pilot project in Kentucky that, with the assistance of the ophthalmic industry, expanded to all 50 states and the District of Columbia by 1991. Today VISION USA is recognized throughout the country by social service agencies and others who work with low-income people as a program that provides eye and vision care to persons in need who are financially ineligible for regular public assistance. Since 1991 VISION USA has provided free eye care to over 262,000 low-income children and adults nationwide. It is an ideal way for doctors of optometry to participate in a coordinated and organized program of community service and care giving for the indigent.

Organized optometry also provides services to the indigent of some communities through the clinics of the schools and colleges of optometry. Although the level of care provided in optometric educational institutions is quite similar to that provided in the private community, teaching clinics typically have lower costs and strong ties to the community. While these institutions may not be able to offer free care, they frequently provide eye and vision care services on a sliding scale, or through some other reduced fee system or extended method of payment. Patients in teaching clinics often invest a significant amount of time rather than money to receive their care, as a supervised optometric student may take much longer than a trained practitioner to provide a comprehensive eye and vision examination. In this way, patients in teaching clinics also make an important contribution to the education of future health care practitioners.

Despite the availability of private charity, there are times when outside financial resources may be unavailable when a specific indigent patient needs care. In such cases the optometrist could provide eye and vision care to needy patients by providing services and materials as a direct contribution, providing care in the office setting at no or reduced cost. For some patients it will be possible to establish a long-term payment plan that respects the individual's financial circumstances and recognizes the value of the optometrist's services. And while the practice of paying for health care through the provision of non-monetary goods or services is no longer as common as it was fifty years ago, there are times when the optometrist may agree to be paid in this way.

Equal Respect for All Patients

For paying and non-paying patients alike — as a point of ethics and good practice management — optometrists must make certain that their offices are friendly and openly welcoming to everyone. Attitudes, language, and subtle behaviors can create the atmosphere that defines an office environment as friendly or unfriendly toward the indigent. Optometrists should be aware of and remove visible and invisible barriers and stigmatizing practices that may interfere with well-intentioned efforts to provide care for the indigent, including inadequate approaches to patient communication. For example, it is always inappropriate for the receptionist to discuss a patient's bill or financial situation within earshot of others in the waiting area or exam rooms. Similarly, staff should not reveal patients' source of payment, and payment status should be considered confidential information not to be discussed with others unless the patient has granted permission to release the information.

Indigent patients should not be asked to participate in research or training activities for which paying patients are not also recruited. It is unethical to perform unnecessary tests or procedures to get practice with a new technique or instrument without full disclosure and consent. Nonetheless, many poor people, particularly members of ethnic minority groups, are fearful that health care professionals will use them for training or experimentation under the guise of providing uncompensated care. One legacy of the Tuskegee Syphilis Study (1932-1972), in which the U.S. Public Health Service denied effective treatment to a group of African American men over a period of forty years, is the persistent concern that health care professionals cannot be trusted to serve the welfare of the poor.[10] Where research or training is conducted, indigent persons may be particularly vulnerable to "manipulative or coercive incentives," such as providing a nominal fee to participate or withholding important information.[11] Fully voluntary informed consent should be obtained before involving the patient in research or educational projects.

In the dispensary, indigent patients should not have to endure the stigma of being singled out for "special" services or products, such as being required to select frames from a special display labeled "Medicaid" or that is brought out only when an indigent patient is selecting a frame. Such practices identify the patient as different, both to the individual and any onlookers. Products, programs, and services designed to help indigent patients should be integrated as much as possible into the mainstream activities of the practice. They should appear seamless to the patient, optometrist, staff, and others in the waiting area.

Irrespective of their ability to pay, patients tend to judge the quality of their care on the basis of how they are treated while in the office, and not on the results of any intervention. A patient's good clinical outcome can easily be jeopardized by poor personal interaction with the optometrist or office staff. Indigent patients should enjoy the same level of attention, concern, and respect as non-indigent patients. They should not feel that they are being treated differently or that they are a burden on the optometrist's time. Appropriate office etiquette can help reduce the apprehension of indigent patients, and build trusting relationships between the optometrist and all patients, irrespective of their financial status.

Ethical principles and values are the foundation of professional integrity. Concern for the patient must be primary, and all other interests, including the optometrist's personal financial welfare, must remain secondary in patient care and clinical decision making. Respect for patients must be consistent and universal, and not dependent on the patient's ability to pay, fluctuations in attitude among office personnel, or other interpersonal variables irrelevant to the principles of clinical ethics. By attending to the needs of the indigent, optometrists can reinforce the profession's commitment to the welfare of all patients and enhance the profession's ethical standing in society.

References

1. Bailey RN. The history of ethics in the American Optometric Association 1898-1994. *J Am Optom Assoc* 1994; 65: 427-44.
2. Bayles MD. Trust and the professional-client relationship. In: Flores A, ed. *Professional ideals*. Belmont, CA: Wadsworth Publishing Co., 1988: 66-80.
3. American College of Physicians. Ethics manual, fourth edition. *Ann Intern Med* 1998; 128: 576-94.
4. Snyder L, ed. *Ethical choices: case studies for medical practice*. Philadelphia, PA: American College of Physicians, 1996.
5. Beauchamp TL, Childress JF. *Principles of biomedical ethics*, 4th ed. New York, Oxford University Press, 1994.
6. Campbell CS, Rogers VC. The normative principles of dental ethics. In: Weinstein BD. *Dental ethics*. Malvern, PA: Lea & Febiger, 1993: 20-41.
7. Ozar DT. Virtues, values, and norms in dentistry. In: Weinstein BD. *Dental ethics*. Malvern, PA: Lea & Febiger, 1993: 3-19.
8. Classé JG. Conflicts of law and ethics in the practice of optometry. *J Am Optom Assoc* 1994; 65: 414-6.
9. Roth MS. That no person shall lack for visual care, regardless of his financial status. *J Am Optom Assoc* 1994; 65: 397-8.
10. Gamble VN. Under the shadow of Tuskegee: African Americans and health care. *Am J Public Health* 1997; 87: 1773-8.
11. Coughlin SS, Soskolne CL, Goodman KW. *Case studies in public health ethics*. Washington, DC: American Public Health Association, 1997.

Chapter Thirteen

Ethics in Low Vision Rehabilitation

Kia B. Eldred, OD
Elizabeth Hoppe, OD, DrPH

Mrs. Grace has slowly been losing her functional vision due to glaucoma for three years. She already has a closed circuit television, bioptic telescopes, and a number of magnifiers, but she rarely uses any of them. Over the two years since she first came to see him, Dr. Peng has been dismayed by Mrs. Grace's lack of goals and her husband's insistence on providing for even her most basic daily living needs. On this visit, however, Mrs. Grace seems despondent: "If I can't read I don't want to go on living," she tells Dr. Peng. Mrs. Grace is accompanied by her adult son, who tells Dr. Peng that his father recently had a stroke and will likely be confined to a wheel chair for the rest of his life. "We could probably afford to keep both my parents at home with a paid attendant," he tells Dr. Peng, "if Mother could qualify for disability benefits."

Optometry is uniquely equipped to work with patients with visual impairments and to interact with other health care professionals in the field of rehabilitation. Rehabilitation typically aims to maximize individuals' functional ability when illness or injury has compromised their physical and/or mental capacities. The diagnosis and treatment of low vision extends beyond patients' visual problems to consideration and concern for the whole person. Individuals with low vision deserve the optometrist's compassion and respect in addition to skillful diagnosis and treatment.

In caring for patients with impaired vision, optometrists must typically balance the ethical principles of beneficence, respect for autonomy, protection of the vulnerable, and truth-telling. The ethical principle of beneficence requires optometrists to place their patients' welfare at the highest level of concern. In almost every aspect of low vision care, the patient must be part of the solution to the problem. The optometrist must respect the patient's autonomy in order for the patient to take an active role. However, the visually impaired can also be especially vulnerable. Many visually impaired patients are elderly and in poor general health. Optometrists may be called to go to greater lengths than usual to protect visually impaired patients and to help preserve their independence and dignity. Because the complexities of the health care system and qualifying for disability benefits can prove very daunting for many patients, optometrists must serve as patient advocates and help their patients receive the best available care. Such advocacy must nonetheless recognize the importance of truthful reporting of examination results, both to patients and, as required, to governmental agencies that provide services and other benefits to patients with visual impairments.

Low Vision and the Definition of "Legally Blind"

The term low vision includes a variety of conditions and degrees of impairment. The American Medical Association has published criteria and methods for evaluating permanent impairments of the visual system and for relating visual impairments to the permanent impairment of the whole person. Evaluation of visual impairment is based on corrected visual acuity for far and near objects, visual field perception, and ocular motility with diplopia. A "percent loss" can be calculated for each eye, then translated into a "percent impairment" for the visual system and the whole person.[1]

When working with patients who are visually impaired, optometrists are asked to act both as caregivers and as agents of the government, authorized to determine who qualifies as legally blind for state or federal agencies. In the United States, legal blindness has been defined as a best corrected distance acuity of 20/200 or worse, or a visual field constricted to a diameter of 20 degrees or less.[2] Best correction refers to conventional spectacle or contact lens correction and does not include the use of telescopes or other low vision devices. The Social Security Act defines legal blindness in the following terms:

> An individual shall be considered to be blind for the purposes of this title if he has central visual acuity of 20/200 or less in the better eye with

the use of a correcting lens. An eye which is accompanied by a limitation in the fields of vision such that the widest diameter of the visual field subtends an angle of no more than 20 degrees shall be considered for purposes of the first sentence of this subsection as having a central visual acuity of 20/200 or less.[3] Classification as legally blind requires an independent determination of disability based on clinical findings.

Individuals who are declared legally blind are eligible for many federal, state, and local social service programs. Social Security Disability Insurance (SSDI) provides supplemental income from the federal government to individuals with a qualified, medically determinable physical or mental impairment. A special provision under Title II extends SSDI benefits to blind workers who have attained the age of 55 and have "the inability, because of blindness, to engage in substantial gainful activity requiring skills or abilities comparable to those of any gainful activity in which he or she has previously engaged."[3] Additionally, the designation of legally blind entitles an individual to an extra exemption when filing federal income tax, access to "talking books" and other audio materials from the Library of Congress, services from state departments of rehabilitation, special transportation services in many cities, and often discounted fares on airlines or trains. It is generally in the interest of an individual with low vision to be declared legally blind in order that they may qualify for these helpful services.

Patients' desire for the benefits that accompany the legal determination of blindness can create difficult practical and ethical questions for optometrists committed both to helping their patients and to reporting their findings as truthfully as possible. Most optometrists specializing in low vision use equipment that improves diagnostic precision, but which may complicate the determination of blindness. For example, the Feinbloom Low Vision Chart presents lines of acuity that are different from those found on the standard Snellen chart. The level of acuity of 20/200 could be claimed for three different lines on the Feinbloom Low Vision Chart (10/60 10/80, and 10/100) as compared to just two letters on the Snellen chart. The Feinbloom chart is also of higher contrast, as it is a printed rather than a projected chart. Optometrists using the Feinbloom chart to determine legal blindness may still need to have patients read the Snellen chart if their level is 10/60 or 10/80, so that blindness can be determined based on the "standard" eye chart.

Another area of concern when certifying patients as legally blind is testing of visual fields. Individuals with advanced retinitis pigmentosa who may have a remaining arc of vision in the periphery may present with only one meridian more than what is required for certification. Whether such patients are legally blind is difficult to answer. The question must be judged on a case-by-case basis, in light of the patient's functional vision level.

Classifying patients who report different levels of performance at different levels of illumination or varying levels of contrast presents another practical and ethical challenge. A patient's lowest level of performance may qualify as blindness whereas his or her highest level would not. Here again, it is important to evaluate the whole person. The most important consideration is the patient's usual setting and whether in day-to-day events their vision problems are significant. Individuals who are functionally impaired the majority of time should be considered eligible for disability status.

Follow-up testing of patients who have been certified to be legally blind may occasionally create ethical questions as well. If follow-up testing concludes that the patient's visual acuity and/or functional vision do not meet the criteria for legal blindness, the legitimacy of the patient's claim of disability may be questioned. Whether the optometrist should report these new results to relevant governmental agencies, potentially revoking the patient's eligibility for benefits, is again a case-by-case decision that depends on the optometrist's interpretation of the meaning of the test results for the patient's overall functional ability.

Rehabilitation and Respect for Autonomy

Whatever the extent of a patient's visual impairment, optometrists working in the area of low vision endeavor to maximize patients' functional ability through rehabilitation. Rehabilitation requires that the patient be involved in treatment and truly desire some functional improvement. Without personal motivation, patients will not be helped by the rehabilitation process. Thus, it is important for the optometrist to work with the low vision patient in identifying the patient's own goals for treatment and how to achieve them.

Setting and working toward functional goals can be difficult for some patients with visual impairments due to the complexity of many diagnoses, and the progressive deterioration that may accompany even the best treatment. The optometrist's first responsibility in helping low vision patients set treatment goals is to be truthful in describing the patient's condition and its probable course, and then to present the patient with the reasonable options for care. Both beneficence and respect for the patient's autonomy require that the optometrist help the patient understand his or her diagnosis as well as the interventions that offer some potential benefit. At times the patient's goals may be different from what the optometrist would suggest, and the patient may want another course of treatment than what the optometrist would recommend. Respect for autonomy means recognizing the patient's right to make his or her own choices. In some instances, this may even mean accepting the patient's choice to "do nothing."

When the patient chooses a course of action that differs significantly from the optometrist's recommendation, it is important to determine why the patient has made this choice and whether it indicates differing values, poor understanding of the disease or treatment options, fear of the condition or the consequences of intervention, or diminished capacity for decision making. The complexity of many of the causes of low vision may require the optometrist to explain the same information in different ways over time before the patient understands his or her condition. Fear of the unknown may prevent some patients from accepting potentially sight-restoring treatment, as in the case of the patient with dense, visually impairing cataracts or the patient with a benign pituitary tumor who is slowly losing all light perception, both of whom may be unduly afraid of surgery.

Many patients also become depressed during the course of their vision loss.[4] A once vital and active person may become morose and despondent when faced with the threat of blindness. Someone who was previously very independent may lose interest in past activities and demand the constant support of family members or friends. Depression usually can be treated with medication or therapy, which may renew the patient's desire for independence and an improved quality of life. Because depression is a real risk for many patients with progressive loss of vision, optometrists need to be able to distinguish depression from patients' other reasons for not seeking intervention or rehabilitative services. Moreover, new low vision patients should be advised that depression may accompany their loss of vision. The optometrist should reassure patients that he or she has resources available for the diagnosis and treatment of depression whenever it may be an issue.

In some instances, as in the case of Dr. Peng and Mrs. Grace, patients with visual impairment may learn to be dependent rather than independent, and functional dependence may become an important part of their personal and family relationships. Such dependence may be the patient's own choice, and he or she may derive some psychological, social, or emotional benefit from the impairment. In such cases it may be difficult to determine why the patient does not respond to rehabilitation without evaluating his or her wider environment. With the patient's consent, family members should be brought in to the discussion of the goals of treatment, and enlisted to help the patient achieve those goals.

While the right to refuse treatment is an important aspect of patient autonomy, optometrists must be able to recognize when the patient is not competent to make his or her own decisions. At times the condition causing the patient's visual impairment may also result in or contribute to incompetence. Patients with such conditions may be at risk of self-neglect. Self-neglect is characterized as the behavior of an individual that threatens his or her own health or safety. Self-neglect may manifest itself dramatically as the patient's refusal or failure to provide him or herself with adequate food, water, clothing, or shelter. It may also be demonstrated as a lack of personal hygiene, refusal of needed medication, or neglect of safety precautions.[4] Among the elderly, who make up a large segment of the population with low vision, self-neglect may constitute a form of elder abuse that the optometrist must report to adult protective services. Determining when self-neglect is a factor in a patient's refusal of low vision services, whether the patient is incompetent to make treatment decisions regarding his or her condition, and whether the patient's situation warrants reporting as elder abuse requires a combination of clinical judgment and ethical insight in each case.

Visually impaired and legally blind children are another potentially vulnerable population whose welfare may be significantly affected by good low vision care. There is some evidence that individuals with congenital visual impairments may not be referred for specialty care as promptly as are those who are diagnosed with an acquired visual impairment.[5] Although some health care professionals may believe that it is not appropriate to refer visually impaired children until they are almost school age and able to use an assistive device, children's needs outside the classroom also deserve attention. Children are very adaptable and are often interested in seeing better even at early ages. Parents of visually impaired children often need information and professional guidance to maximize their child's abilities and learning potential, and both parents and children benefit most when they receive needed information early in the child's life.

It can also be extremely important to identify children's visual impairments before their conditions are misinterpreted by others. Developmental or intelligence tests that include a visual component, which are commonly used in elementary schools, may falsely identify children with visual problems as developmentally delayed or mentally handicapped. It can be quite difficult to "unlabel" a child wrongly categorized by standardized intelligence tests, even after a comprehensive eye and vision assessment has identified the real problem.

Children who are both physically and mentally handicapped may often be affected by visual impairments that go undetected because of their other problems. For such children objective vision testing is an important part of an overall functional assessment. However, objective testing alone is not enough to assist these patients. It is important that they be examined as thoroughly as possible, and referred to an appropriate low vision specialist for evaluation if the correct equipment is not available. Spectacles should be suggested when necessary, even for children whose lives are very limited functionally, as addressing visual problems may contribute to the child's development in other areas and enhance his or her practical independence.

Promoting Patients' Independence and Protecting the Public's Safety: Driving Issues

In today's society, functional independence often requires the ability to drive a car. The issue of driving with a visual impairment is quite controversial. Low vision patients may ask for optical devices that would allow them to qualify for a driver's license. Such requests may create serious ethical dilemmas for optometrists, who have important obligations to protect public safety as well as responsibilities to their individual patients. A patient who may qualify for a driver's license with an assistive device may still not see well enough to be a safe driver.

If a patient falls within the legal guidelines for driving and asks to be fitted with an assistive device, the optometrist must weigh his or her responsibilities to the public as well as patient autonomy. Driving is a privilege, not a right, and optometrists must be concerned with the safety of the patient as well as that of others. It is ultimately the state that makes the final decision regarding the patient's ability to drive. The laws in each state differ in regard to eligibility for visually impaired drivers, and there is no authoritative study that definitively states what visual field size or visual acuity level is truly safe.

Visual field testing is not required prior to licensure in most states, yet visual fields may be a more important parameter than visual acuity when driving.[6] Most state licensing agencies appear to assume that if central vision is normal then peripheral vision is normal. The size of the visual field for driving is often stated in testing handbooks, but parameters are not mentioned for the testing of visual fields. In some states, drivers with no tickets and no previously documented health condition that might affect their driving may be given the option of renewing their driver's license by mail. In these situations neither visual acuity nor visual field is tested, and individuals with significantly impaired vision may not be identified prior to the renewal of their licenses.

Moreover, other variables involved with driving, such as judgment, reflexes, physical ability, etc., are just as important as the visual requirements, if not more so. Even if the optometrist believes that a patient would not be able to pass the road test of the driving exam, he or she is not qualified to assess a patient's abilities in these other areas. Nonetheless, optometrists are often in a position to encourage or discourage a patient from pursuing a license, and may be compelled to report a patient's impairment to the state. The limited nature of most states' driver's license vision tests creates ethical problems for optometrists who believe that certain patients should not be given a driver's license, or who learn that patients with progressive vision loss are still driving even after their vision becomes dangerously low. Whether to report a licensed driver who has passed the visual portion of the driver's test but whose visual field is smaller than required by the state regulations is just one such example.

When an optometrist does fit a patient with a bioptic device to enable the patient to drive, he or she is obviously obliged to determine the patient's best acuity and visual field with the device. In addition, however, eye movements and scanning ability have a great deal to do with successful driving, and the ability to use the bioptic device appropriately is essential. It is not enough simply to prescribe the device and send the patient for a road test. No one will be prepared to drive with an assistive device without some degree of instruction and practice, and optometrists should refer patients for such training before they attempt to use a device to pass the driver's license exam.

Despite the importance of respect for autonomy, the optometrist should recognize when low-vision patients forfeit the right to drive because their driving may put the public at risk. Optometrists who believe that a patient poses a threat to others when he or she gets behind the wheel of a car may have a duty to report their professional opinion and relevant information to the police or other governmental agency. However, only some states mandate the reporting of patients whose vision does not qualify them to drive, and a breach of a confidentiality where reporting is not required may put the optometrist at risk of legal action by the patient. To the extent possible, optometrists should work closely with their low vision patients to help them evaluate their own need and ability to drive. When patients are unable to drive, the optometrist can help plan other forms of transportation that will maximize their independent mobility without compromising public safety.

Confidentiality of Information

Beyond the potential interest of driver's licensing authorities in the visual impairments of optometrists' low vision patients, other individuals and organizations may seek information about the extent and implications of an individual's vision problems. The American Optometric Association (AOA) Code of Ethics declares that optometrists "hold in professional confidence all information concerning a patient and to use such data only for the benefit of the patient." Thus the optometrist must be able to protect patients' confidentiality while, as requested, explaining his or her visual impairments to others.

For example, employers have many reasons to be concerned about the vision of their employees. Not only may individuals' visual impairment affect the quality of their work, it may also affect their ability to do certain jobs safely. Since the passage of the Americans with Disabilities Act (ADA), employers are required to make reasonable accommodations for employees with disabilities.[7] Optometrists may be asked to provide information related to low vision patients' job qualifications and performance in order for their employers to make accommodations for their disability. However, patients may also ask their optometrists for help in concealing their visual impairment from employers and others when their impairments are not relevant to the job.

Family members may also want information about relatives' vision loss or impairment. Family support is an essential part of rehabilitation. Most low vision patients will need their family's encouragement and assistance, and elderly patients must often rely on younger family members who need information about their parent's or relative's visual status in order to provide meaningful help. However, protecting the confidentiality and welfare of elderly patients, in particular, often means understanding the relationship between older patients and their adult children. There are patients who do not want other family members to know about their visual impairment, even when they need family members' help to cope with the consequences of low vision.

Additionally, many partially sighted patients have a genetic or hereditary eye disease as the cause of their impairment. Whether to disclose the patient's diagnosis and information about genetic transmission with his or her spouse, children, or other relatives again poses the ethical challenge of balancing respect for the patient's autonomy and privacy with concern for the welfare of others affected by the patient's condition. The specific genes for juvenile-onset primary open-angle glaucoma, retinitis pigmentosa, and age-related macular degeneration have all been identified.[8] Testing for a genetic marker for an ocular disease that may not manifest until much later in life, such as macular degeneration, may permit affected individuals to plan for their later disability and free unaffected individuals from years of worry. However, disclosing patients' genetic conditions to others, even to family members, may expose them to potential psychological harm and social stigma that the optometrist is likely unprepared to address.[8] Generally neither a patient's employer nor family members has "a right to know" information about his or her visual impairments, its causes, treatment, or likely prognosis without the patient's consent.

Access to Low Vision Rehabilitation Services

Despite the benefits of specialized optometric care for patients with low vision, patients with ocular pathologies are often not referred for low vision services or told about the types of vision rehabilitation care that might be available. Research in one low vision center found that patients were delayed an average of nearly six years from the time of diagnosis to the first low vision service.[5] Many patients ask in their first low vision examination, "Why didn't anyone tell me that this was available?"

The AOA Code of Ethics states that optometrists are "to advise the patient whenever consultation with an optometric colleague or reference for other professional care seems advisable." Supporting the need to refer patients for vision rehabilitation are the guiding ethical principles of beneficence and collegiality. Optometrists should refer for low vision services any patients who are experiencing functional vision loss if they choose not to provide these services themselves. Referral is necessary regardless of the patient's level of visual acuity, because one patient may experience impairment at the level of 20/40, where another has no difficulty at the level of 20/80. Patients whose goals cannot be achieved with the devices and services available in one optometrist's practice should be referred to an office that can better meet the needs of the patient. Referral may be to address one specific goal, after which the patient will return to the original optometrist, or it may entail a complete transfer of care so that all the goals of the patient can be met.

When referring a patient for low vision services, it is helpful for the referring doctor to provide as comprehensive information as possible regarding the patient's condition and previous examination findings. If proper information is not provided, examination services may be duplicated by the low vision specialist, requiring additional professional time and resulting in unnecessary expense. In addition, the low vision specialist will likely have difficulty discussing the patient's prognosis if full referral information has not been made available. Ethical difficulties may also arise in coding and billing for patients who are improperly referred for low vision services if it is subsequently determined that they needed only a more refined refraction.

Comprehensive vision rehabilitation services may be costly, and assistive devices can be a considerable expense for many patients with visual impairments. Preventing the costs of low vision services from becoming a barrier to access to care is a significant practical and ethical challenge for optometrists. Many specialists in low vision work in not-for-profit clinics that serve large numbers of patients with limited incomes. Often such clinics set the price of diagnostic testing and prescribed devices on a sliding scale that permits access for insured and uninsured patients at varying income levels. Private practitioners, however, may not be able to charge less for assistive devices without absorbing significant financial cost themselves. Optometrists in such situations should note the precept of the AOA's Code of Ethics that none shall lack for optometric care regardless of financial status, and may consider referring some patients to less expensive not-for-profit clinics. Moreover, they must also work to ensure that low vision patients do not refuse beneficial interventions and sacrifice improved functional ability out of concern for cost.

While some patients refuse potentially life-changing interventions because of cost, others may spend thousands of dollars pursuing treatments of questionable value. Part of the patient's psychological adaptation to loss of vision and one of the expected stages of loss includes "searching for a cure."[9] Optometrists who practice in the field of low vision may receive general requests from patients for the latest alleged breakthrough or specific inquiries about an experimental intervention that may have been reported in the news media. Some of these therapeutic approaches may be controversial, such as the use of thalidomide for treatment of macular degeneration.[10] Others may be unproven "natural" or herbal interventions popularized by lay health publications and Internet sites. Some interventions may also be potentially dangerous to the ocular or systemic health of the patient, such as large doses of certain vitamins and minerals.[11] Optometrists should keep abreast of the news on "breakthrough" treatments, carefully weigh the evidence presented in current scientific literature, and beware of unvalidated claims. Professional opinion should be informed, even if there is no preponderance of evidence on either side.

The practice of low vision rehabilitation requires the willingness to work with patients whose lives have been devastated by a loss of vision. Their care demands compassion and patience with the slow and deliberate pace of treatment, as well as the ability to celebrate small improvements of vision when complete restoration of sight cannot be expected. The challenges of low vision care are often matched by the rewards of interacting with patients who value their remaining vision tremendously and who consider optometrists their indispensable allies in the struggle to protect it.

Acknowledgment: The authors gratefully acknowledge the helpful comments of Alfred Rosenbloom, OD, of The Chicago Lighthouse, Chicago, IL.

References

1. American Medical Association. *Guide to the evaluation of permanent impairment,* 4th ed. Chicago, IL: AMA, 1993.
2. Social Security Act of 1935 Sec. 216 [42 USC 416] i(1)(B).

3. Social Security Act of 1935 Sec. 1614 [42 USC 1382c] a(2).

4. Emerson DL. Adjusting to visual impairment. In: Faye EE, ed. *Clinical low vision.* Boston, MA: Little, Brown, & Co. Inc., 1984: 379-88.

5. Hoppe E, Bowyer NK, Evans S. Access to vision rehabilitation services for older adults. Presented at the American Academy of Optometry Annual Meeting, Orlando, FL, December 1992.

6. Shipp MD. Potential human and economic cost-savings attributable to vision testing policies for driver license renewal, 1989-1991. *Optom Vision Sci* 1998; 75(2): 103-18.

7. U.S. Equal Employment Opportunity Commission and U.S. Department of Justice. *Americans with Disabilities Act Handbook.* Washington, DC: U.S. Government Printing Office, 1992.

8. Wormington C. The Human Genome Project. Presented at the American Academy of Optometry Annual Meeting, San Francisco, CA, December 1998.

9. Faye EE. Preface. In: Faye EE, ed. *Clinical low vision.* Boston, MA: Little, Brown, & Co. Inc., 1984: xi-xiii.

10. Ip M, Gorin MB. Recurrence of a choroidal neovascular membrane in a patient with punctate inner choroidopathy treated with daily doses of thalidomide. *Am J Ophthalmol* 1996; 122: 594-5.

11. Beiting J. Will a vitamin a day keep eye disease away? http://www.eye-world.org

Chapter Fourteen

Clinical Optometry in a Multicultural Society

Elizabeth Heitman, PhD
Siu G. Wong, OD

Dr. Carroll looked at the boy, and then at the man who had just sat down in the exam chair. The man nudged the boy. "Díle a la doctora que se me arañó el ojo ayer y que me duele. Y díle que se me quebraron los lentes y que necesito otros."* The child turned to the optometrist and said shyly, "My grandfather wants glasses." Dr. Carroll had taken Spanish in high school but found it hard to work with the growing number of Spanish-speaking patients who came to her office. She was glad to see that this patient had brought his 9-year-old grandson to translate.

Across the United States, optometrists are challenged to meet the needs of patients whose expectations and experience of optometry are shaped by cultural factors foreign to the provider. As immigration makes the U.S. population more ethnically diverse, both optometrists and their patients are influenced by a broader spectrum of cultural characteristics than ever before. When the cultural backgrounds of the optometrist and patient are different, it is especially important for them to communicate about their beliefs and expectations, but communication may be significantly hampered by their cultural differences. Where communication is difficult, especially where the optometrist and patient speak different languages, trust becomes simultaneously more important and more difficult to sustain. Because even minor cultural differences may result in ethical conflict and the disruption of care, optometrists must pay special attention to cultural issues across their practices.

---

*"Tell the doctor that I scratched my eye yesterday and that it hurts. And tell her that I broke my glasses and need new ones."

Culture and Health Care

Culture is a universal factor of human life, but is something that few people can define easily. Race, language, nationality, geographic origin, and religious belief are important aspects of culture, but their expression may vary a great deal among groups and individuals claiming the same cultural background. In much of the professional literature on culture and health care, cultural issues are often discussed in relation to ethnic minority patients. Clearly, ethnic minority patients' cultural beliefs, socio-economic status, and English proficiency affect both their health and their access to health care. However, there is also growing cultural diversity among health professionals, including practitioners trained abroad and first-generation Americans who pursue careers in health care. To some extent, the scientific orientation of professional education limits the effects of caregivers' personal cultural heritage on the treatment that they provide. However, caregivers' cultural presuppositions about the social roles and behavior of different groups often persist despite their technical training.

Many people do not recognize their own culturally shaped beliefs and behaviors, and many cultural factors in health care become apparent only when there is conflict between the patient's and practitioner's expectations or actions. Irrespective of the backgrounds of optometrists and patients, culturally based beliefs and assumptions shape their perspectives on eye and vision care in four important areas: the definition of health and illness, the nature of appropriate treatment, the role of the patient, and the role of the health care provider.

Health and illness

In most societies, "health" is typically defined in terms of what is normal, and "illness" in terms of what is abnormal. As a result, even a condition that causes significant impairment may not be treated as an illness in populations where the problem is prevalent. For example, cataracts were once considered a normal part of old age. Health care practitioners identify specific diseases based on the presence of certain symptoms and signs.

Certain cultural groups are more likely to experience certain conditions than are others, due to genetic predisposition, environmental factors, and/or cultural practices. However, the way in which symptoms are categorized and linked with particular illnesses is also strongly affected by culture. In one review of the World Health Organization (WHO) International Classification of Diseases, only slightly more than half were found to be recognized conditions in the U.S. health care system — the rest were what is known as "culture bound syndromes," in which groups of symptoms are interpreted in light of important cultural themes and values.[1] For example, the condition known throughout the non-western world as "evil eye" has symptoms similar to those of depression, but its cause is said to be another person's jealousy or an evil spirit's envy of human beauty or happiness.[2]

Even where a disease is recognized across cultures, the explanation of symptoms and their causes may vary with culture: for example, traditional Chinese medicine holds that swollen, red, and teary eyes reflect a liver disorder.[3] Descriptions of illness and specific symptoms may also vary among cultural groups. Some languages may even not have words for relatively common conditions; for example, there is no word for virus in Hindi. In contrast, some cultures may have health-related concepts that cannot be expressed easily in English, such as the yin and yang forces that are essential to the Asian view of health and illness.[3] The optometrist's ability to diagnose a patient's condition appropriately will depend on his or her ability to recognize the cultural boundaries of all definitions of health, illness, and particular conditions.

Appropriate treatment

Patients want treatment that fits with their understanding of their condition and what has caused it. For example, an Asian patient with puffy, red, and teary eyes who accepted the Chinese medicine's traditional link between the eyes and internal organs might be unsatisfied with topical antibiotic drops intended to treat conjunctivitis. Additionally, patients from different cultural groups may prefer different forms of treatment for the same condition. Patients may even reject effective treatment if it does not match the logic of their culture's definition of health and illness or preferred method of intervention. In cross-cultural patient care, successful treatment depends both on the optometrist's ability to determine what patients think they need and why, and ability to help patients understand recommended interventions in a way that fits with their cultural beliefs.

The patient's role

In the ethics of the contemporary U.S. health care system, the individual patient is considered to be the focus of attention. However, in societies where individuality is not as important a value as it is in the United States, disease is understood to affect families and communities as well as individual family members. In traditional African, Hispanic, Asian, and European families, the patient with physical symptoms may be accompanied to the optometrist's office by one or more family members who believe that family interests are at stake in the proper diagnosis and treatment of the patient's condition. To work effectively with such patients, it is important for the optometrist to know whether the patient and family expect the focus of intervention to be the individual with the physical symptoms, the family in which the condition occurs, or even the community affected by the infirmity of its members.

Optometry generally accepts the U.S. health care system's definition of the patient's role, which emphasizes self-determination and the patient's individual interaction with the optometrist who provides his or her eye and vision care. However, the concept of patient autonomy common in the United States is foreign to many cultures, both non-western and European. Instead, the family often takes over the sick person's responsibilities, including speaking for the patient, in recognition of his or her condition. U.S. optometrists' efforts to include their patients in decision making may be rejected by families accustomed to other cultural practices that support withholding information or lying to loved ones about serious illness. The U.S. legal requirement that patients sign a consent document prior to certain procedures may pose an even greater problem, especially for patients and families from non-literate societies where signing formal documents implies that something monumental is about to occur.

The practitioner's role

At the outset, the patient or patient's family defines the practitioner's role in diagnosis and treatment by the simple act of choosing whom to ask for help. Most people, whatever their cultural background, do not seek professional assistance immediately after determining that they have a health problem, unless it is acute or painful. In many immigrant communities this delay is often due to specific barriers to access to care, such as the unavailability of practitioners in the area, the patient's limited ability to speak English, and the patient's inability to afford health care. Patients' uncertainty about the expertise of different health care professions may also affect their use of optometrists relative to other health care professionals. This confusion is due in part to the many different scopes of practice worldwide and the different requirements for professional education leading to the title optometrist.[4] For example, the direct translation of optometrist in Cantonese is "fix the eyeglasses doctor," and Cantonese patients may not seek an optometrist's care for more comprehensive eye and vision care. In some countries, the title optometrist is used by individuals who make glasses using little more than an auto-refractor to obtain the patient's prescription. In a related area, Spanish-speaking patients may not know what services to expect when they visit the optometrist for screening or a comprehensive examination, as the term "screening" has no direct Spanish equivalent and "examination" may be used in both senses.

Once the patient is in the optometrist's office, how he or she will respond to the individual practitioner may depend on culturally influenced interpretations of authority and trustworthiness. In traditional societies, an older optometrist would likely be respected because of the presumed wisdom that accompanies age, whereas in the technologically oriented United States, people often assume that a younger clinician will have more recent knowledge and better technical skills than an older practitioner. Similarly, whereas the number of women in optometry in the United States is rapidly increasing, among patients whose cultures reinforce traditional gender roles, a woman optometrist may be presumed at first to be a technician or assistant to a male doctor. The "right" appearance is also important to authority and trustworthiness — whether that means wearing a white laboratory coat, a suit or skirt, or more casual office clothing, the optometrist who does not look the part to some patients may not be acceptable to them, regardless of his or her actual abilities.

Communication and Patient Care

Wherever the expectations of optometrists and their patients differ, there is a real possibility of miscommunication and conflict, leading to a poor outcome for the patient and the failure of the interaction generally. To prevent differences in culturally based definitions from affecting the patient's care – or to address problems that have already occurred – it is important for the optometrist to recognize that there is a cultural difference between them. Only then will it be possible to identify the conflicting culturally based expectations and engage the patient in discussion that can negotiate a workable compromise.

However, communication itself is affected by culture.[5] A caring and concerned optometrist may give patients a very different impression if he or she is unaware of how efforts to communicate may be interpreted through other cultural lenses. The direct language that many U.S. clinicians are taught to use in asking questions and describing a patient's condition and proposed treatment may seem shockingly abrupt to many people of non-western backgrounds. In contrast, asking vague open-ended questions, such as "how is your vision" may be misinterpreted by both direct speakers and those who value indirect communication.

Similarly, both the volume and pitch with which the optometrist and patient speak may be presumed by the other to indicate the absence or presence of honesty, anger, intelligence, and compassion. And unfortunately, even when the optometrist and patient use the right words at the right pace and tone of voice, a regional or national accent may trigger prejudicial assumptions that complicate their interaction.

Moreover, communication goes beyond spoken words. Misunderstandings and even conflict may result over different interpretations of specific body language and behaviors that are often subtle and unconscious. Hispanic, Asian, and Native American patients may avoid direct eye contact as a sign of respect, which the optometrist may mistake for dishonesty, shame, or fear. Some Navajo and other Native American patients are likely to interpret direct eye contact as a sign that the optometrist is angry or that he or she is challenging them.

Many Asian and Eastern European patients believe that a practitioner's serious demeanor is a sign of concern for the patient's health, and would avoid an optometrist who seemed too enthusiastic or jovial. Both the dimensions of an individual's personal space and the acceptance of gestures and touching vary tremendously across cultures, and if misjudged can convey unintended messages about respect, power, fear, personal concern, and sexuality that can sabotage otherwise good optometric care.

Language Barriers in Clinical Optometry

Clearly, the most difficult challenge to communication occurs when the patient and optometrist do not speak a common language. Language barriers between non-English speaking patients and English speaking health care professionals limit the patients' ability to ask for help and the optometrists' ability to make a diagnosis and provide appropriate care. At a minimum, the optometrist should be able to identify patients who cannot speak English and have a plan for providing appropriate care when such circumstances arise. The ethical standard of care, and increasingly the legal standard as well, is that if something is important enough to communicate about with patients who speak English, it is equally important to discuss with patients who do not speak English, and to do so comprehensibly in the patient's own language.[6]

As U.S. society has become more culturally diverse and fluency in other languages has become more highly valued, the number of bilingual optometrists has increased. Increasing numbers of optometrists, especially among recent graduates of optometry school, are capable of conducting a history and examination in the language spoken by many of their non-English speaking patients. Bilingual optometrists are an important resource for immigrant communities, and many provide an important service to their patients by helping them navigate through the English speaking health care system. However, it is impossible for any practitioner to speak every language that potential patients may speak, especially in larger cities where immigrant communities are in constant flux. Thus, even bilingual optometrists need a plan for working with non-English speaking patients and access to staff or others whose language skills can be counted on when a patient needs an interpreter.

Translating and Interpreters in Clinical Practice

The goal for communication with non-English speaking patients is to achieve the level of meaningful interaction that is the standard of care for English speaking patients. The ideal interpreter should speak the languages of both the patient and the optometrist well. The interpreter must be able to convey the meaning, underlying concepts, and emotional tone of each person's statements and questions to the other, without moral judgment. At times this may mean that the interpreter must explain information as well as translate what is said — however, the interpreter's goal should be to facilitate the relationship between the optometrist and the patient, not to be an advocate or a caregiver or a counselor. Moreover, because interpreters serve as an extension of the optometrist, they are bound by the same ethical commitments to confidentiality and avoiding harm as the optometrist.

This kind of clinical translation requires a high level of skill, knowledge, and commitment to patient welfare, and demands professionalism from the interpreter and a high level of respect from the optometrist. To safeguard the professional standards of their practice, optometrists who have a significant non-English speaking patient population that speaks only a particular language should employ one or more bilingual staff members whose duties officially include interpreting. Ultimately it is the optometrist's responsibility to ensure that such staff perform competently and in the patient's best interest. Because the optometrist may not be able to assess how well the employee actually interprets unless he or she is also bilingual, it is essential that an external authority verify the staff person's fluency. Moreover, the ability to speak another language does not necessarily imply the ability to interpret detailed or sensitive health-related information and advice. Thus, it is vital for the optometrist to provide basic training to bilingual staff in the principles and practice of history taking, interviewing, patient education and counseling, and giving difficult news.

On a practical level, it can be helpful for the optometrist and interpreter to review the non-English speaking patient's record together before the consultation in order to permit the interpreter to check necessary words or phrases, and to prepare for difficult or detailed translations. When an interpreter is used to communicate with a non-English speaking patient, the fact that the interaction was interpreted, as well as the name of the interpreter, should be included in the relevant patient records. Ultimately the interpreter should be able to support the optometrist's report that the non-English speaking patient's treatment met the standard of care, and that essential disclosures and advice were given in a language and format that the patient understood.

Because of the unpredictability of the need for translation, many people who may speak another language besides English are commonly used as interpreters for non-English speaking patients, despite their lack of formal training in translation or optometry, or familiarity with the ethics of patient care. Building maintenance staff, other patients, and patients' family members and friends may be asked to translate patients' clinical information because they are available when the non-English speaking patient comes in. While many of these people are convenient to use, and may seem willing to help when the need for translation arises, their use may create dangerous uncertainties and practical problems during the consultation and afterward.

Most importantly, if the optometrist does not know the person providing translation, it is impossible not only to know how well he or she speaks the patient's language, but more basically how well he or she understands the optometrist's English and the information to be translated. By using a person of unknown language proficiency to provide interpreting, the optometrist is at risk for taking an incomplete or inaccurate history as well as passing on incomplete or inaccurate information to the patient. Even if translation is provided by a well-intentioned lay person, there is a risk for harm to the patient if erroneous or incomplete information is exchanged.

Moreover, if translation is provided by someone whom the patient does not trust, whether a staff member, fellow patient, or family member, the patient may withhold information or lie out of desire for privacy. Having friends or family members translate does not eliminate the concern for confidentiality, as patients may be particularly motivated to protect themselves and their loved ones from the disclosure of sensitive information. Friends and family members, too, may withhold information from patients out of a desire to protect them from unpleasant news, or they may answer the optometrist's questions themselves, based on their own knowledge and perspectives.

The common practice of using bilingual children to translate for their older relatives, as illustrated by the case of Dr. Carroll, also gives undue responsibility to a minor who would not otherwise be considered capable of taking part in such discussion. Additionally, serving as a translator imposes authority on a child to convey questions and information that the patient's culture may consider inappropriate or even rude when directed to an elder. Not only may harm come to the patient from using a child to translate, the child may suffer harm as well.

To prevent as many of the practical and ethical problems involved in clinical interpreting as possible, it is ideal for non-English speaking patients to be scheduled sufficiently far in advance for the optometrist to make suitable arrangements to have an appropriate interpreter available. In large cities it may be possible to call a consulate for assistance in providing language assistance; additionally, some religious and social service organizations can provide occasional interpreters who are familiar with health care terminology and the general ethics of patient care. At other times, it may be necessary to use telephone-based translation services, such as those provided by a number of for-profit agencies. Whenever it is necessary to provide translation by telephone, it is always preferable to use a speaker phone rather than a handset so that everyone can hear what each party says. Even if they do not understand it fully, everyone hearing the full conversation reduces the suspicion that important information is being discussed but not translated, and enhances the mutual trust that is essential to successful care.

Good communication is a cornerstone of good patient care, whatever the cultural backgrounds of the optometrist and patient. As cultural diversity is projected to increase across the U.S. population in the coming years, optometry's continued success will depend on its incorporation of cultural knowledge into the profession's clinical expertise. Where optometrists make a concerted effort to communicate well with all patients, cultural differences may enrich their individual relationships and the profession as a whole.

Acknowledgment: Thanks to Indian Health Service optometrists Richard Hatch, OD, Gallup, NM, and Gary Pabalis, OD, Ft. Duschene, UT for their suggestions.

References

1. Janzen JM. *The quest for therapy: medical pluralism in lower Zaire.* Berkeley, CA: University of California Press, 1978.
2. Galanti G-A. *Caring for patients from different cultures: case studies from American hospitals.* Philadelphia, PA: University of Pennsylvania Press, 1991.
3. Kaptchuk TJ. *The web that has no weaver: understanding Chinese medicine.* New York: Congdon & Weed, 1983.
4. World Council of Optometry. Constitution. Philadelphia, PA: WCO, April 25, 1997.
5. Rogers EM, Steinfatt TM. *Intercultural communication.* Prospect Heights, IL: Waveland Press, Inc., 1999.
6. Perkins J, Simon H, Cheng F, Olson K, Vera Y. *Ensuring linguistic access in health care settings: legal rights and responsibilities.* New York: Henry J. Kaiser Family Foundation, 1998.

Glossary

Assent   Agreement, particularly to a health care intervention, based on as full an understanding and reasoning as possible, that falls short of the standards of consent because of the patient's minor age or mental incapacity.

Autonomy   Self-determination; the ethical principle of respect for autonomy holds that the caregiver must respect patients' right to determine their own interests and make their own choices.

Beneficence   Doing good for and to others; the ethical principle of beneficence in health care holds that the practitioner's professional activities should help those served.

Coercion   Compulsion, restraint, or domination by force or threat.

Collegiality   The mutual support and sharing of authority among persons of similar professional expertise and practice.

Competence   The necessary abilities and capacities for a particular activity; mental ability to make one's own decisions with an appropriate understanding of their consequences.

Confidentiality   Privacy or secrecy, especially of personal or intimate information; the principle of confidentiality holds that health care practitioners will protect patients' confidences and not divulge information obtained from patients except when doing so serves the patients' interests or where required by law to serve imperative public health concerns.

Dignity   Self-worth; characteristic worthy of respect or honor.

Dilemma   A choice between two equally compelling or equally unsatisfactory alternatives, where either option requires a compromise of important values.

Disability   A physical or mental impairment that prevents one from engaging in work or other activities of daily living.

Duty　Tasks, activities, or functions expected or morally required as a result of one's position or role in a group or in society.

Ethical　Related to thoughtful application of values, standards, principles, and theories of right and wrong conduct; consistent with values, standards, principles, and theories that support right conduct.

Ethics　A system of values, standards, principles, and theories that guide or should guide human behavior; systematic reflection on these values, standards, principles, and theories and how they can guide human behavior.

Fiduciary　Relating to, dependent upon, or involving trust or confidence.

Futility　Inability to provide therapeutic benefit or lead to a desired outcome.

Incompetence　Lack of the necessary abilities and capacities to reason and understand, especially with regard to decision making and the consequences of choices or actions.

Informed consent　The process of discussion about proposed health care interventions, in which the practitioner provides information about the procedure's benefits, risks, and alternatives, enabling the patient to make a reasoned decision whether to accept it; also the patient's decision to undergo a proposed treatment after such a discussion.

Justice　Fairness; treating similar cases similarly and ensuring that differences in treatment are related to meaningful differences among cases.

Moral　Related to values and related standards of right and wrong conduct; consistent with values and standards of right conduct.

Morals　Values and related standards of right and wrong conduct that guide or should guide human behavior.

Nonmaleficence   Ethical principle of avoiding doing harm to others, expressed in the classic Hippocratic phrase "primum non nocere" – first do no harm.

Paternalism   The view that health care professionals should make decisions for their patients, based on the model of the father-child relationship where the father has the knowledge and authority to make decisions on behalf of the child.

Placebo effect   The beneficial effect that comes from believing that a treatment will be beneficial; named after the placebo, a pill or other treatment that has no active ingredient or other identified action on the condition for which it is prescribed.

Primum non nocere   Latin for "first do no harm," the classic Hippocratic ethical principle of nonmaleficence.

Principle   A comprehensive or fundamental rule or assumption; the central principles of ethics related to health care include respect for autonomy, beneficence, nonmaleficence, justice, and confidentiality.

Profession   A vocation requiring both specialized training in a distinct area of expertise needed by society and a public commitment to service, which together give the profession independent authority and the responsibility for self-regulation according to high ethical standards.

Professional   A member of one of the professions; related to or consistent with the high ethical standards associated with the professions.

Respect   Consideration, high regard, or esteem based on inherent characteristics of the person or thing valued.

Rights   Claims that one may legitimately expect to be respected or honored by others, including claims to be from others' interference and claims to specific goods, services, or assistance from others.

Standard   An established, authoritative measure or criterion for action or behavior; standards of care may be established through law or professional consensus.

Trust   Confidence in or reliance on the character, ability, or strength of someone or something.

Values   Ideals or principles that reflect beliefs about the meaning and intrinsic worth of people, things, activities, relationships, and institutions.

Appendix

Selected Resolutions of the American Optometric Association House of Delegates Related to Clinical Ethics

The following AOA House of Delegates resolutions are included here as background material due to their implications for the ethical care of patients in the clinical setting, especially in those areas addressed by the chapters of this book. This list does not include all AOA resolutions that may relate to the ethical practice of optometry.

---

769   RELATIONSHIP WITH OPHTHALMOLOGY
(25 of 1947)
(Mod. 1985)   WHEREAS, it is in the best interests of the public that a
                closer relationship exist between ophthalmology and
                optometry; now therefore be it

                RESOLVED, that the profession of optometry is requested to
                continue its efforts in seeking a closer cooperation with oph-
                thalmology for the benefit of the visual welfare of the public.

1883   STANDING COMMITTEE DEALING WITH ETHICS
(2 of 1991)   AND VALUES OF OPTOMETRIC CARE AND SERVICES

                WHEREAS, the profession of optometry has undergone
                dramatic changes in the last half century, including those
                that relate to its scope and organization of practice; and

WHEREAS, the current Code of Ethics of the American Optometric Association was adopted in June of 1944; and

WHEREAS, major clinical pressures and social conditions now prevail which did not exist at that time; now therefore be it

RESOLVED, that the American Optometric Association Board of Trustees establish a standing committee dealing with ethics and values of optometric care and services with a broad mission and focus to address a variety of circumstances and problems which now exist in the health care arena that affect the practices and services of Doctors of Optometry; and be it further

RESOLVED, that the standing committee dealing with ethics and values of optometric care and services make an annual report to the American Optometric Association House of Delegates.

1886   PATIENT CARE DECISIONS INVOLVING
(5 of 1991) THE PRESCRIBING AND DISPENSING OF
(Mod. 1995) OPHTHALMIC PRODUCTS

WHEREAS, patient care decisions involving the prescribing and/or dispensing of ophthalmic products should be made solely on the basis of an eye care provider's professional judgment that is in the patient's best interest; and

WHEREAS, patient care decisions should not be made on the basis of an eye care provider's participation in a manufacturer's advertising and/or promotional program involving the prospect of personal inducements to the eye care provider from a manufacturer; now therefore be it

RESOLVED, that the American Optometric Association opposes any prescribing and/or dispensing of ophthalmic products based on the participation by the eye care provider in a manufacturer's advertising and/or promotional program involving the prospect of personal inducements to the eye care provider from manufacturers.

1890 (9 of 1991)	**HUMAN IMMUNODEFICIENCY VIRUS (HIV) INFECTION**

WHEREAS, the American Optometric Association has, in its 1944 Code of Ethics, held that all patients should be professionally cared for regardless of their personal problems; and

WHEREAS, the Optometric Oath repeats this fundamental principle of ethical concern for the patient; and

WHEREAS, new clinical circumstances in health care of the American public require newer levels of concern for the care of patients with infectious and/or communicable disease; now therefore be it

RESOLVED, that the American Optometric Association in Congress assembled reiterates its time-honored principle of professional care for all patients; and be it further

RESOLVED, that the American Optometric Association strongly recommends that it be the responsibility of all practicing optometrists to acquire background and knowledge, through continuing professional education, of Human Immunodeficiency Virus infections, appropriate infection control and related public health and patient care issues.

1893 (3 of 1992) (Mod. 1995)	**TESTING PRACTITIONERS FOR TUBERCULOSIS**

WHEREAS, the nation is experiencing a serious public health emergency as a result of the resurgence of tuberculosis, an airborne infectious disease; and

WHEREAS, there has been a reappearance of tuberculosis including new highly drug resistant strains; and

WHEREAS, optometrists daily come in close contact with their patients in the course of their examination procedures; now therefore be it

RESOLVED, that the American Optometric Association, as an issue of ethical concern and good public health practice, recommends that all doctors of optometry and their staff have physical examinations at appropriate intervals and an annual test for tuberculosis; and be it further

RESOLVED, that this recommendation includes faculty members at the clinics of the schools and colleges of optometry, and students entering the clinical training phase of their professional education.

1897   CHILD ABUSE

(2 of 1993)   WHEREAS, child abuse is a problem which affects a broad spectrum of the population; and

WHEREAS, there is a need for increased awareness of the physical, psychological and social harm caused by child abuse; and

WHEREAS, doctors of optometry, as primary care providers, are concerned with the physical, behavioral and social aspects of children and may recognize evidence of child abuse in the course of patient care; now therefore be it

RESOLVED, that the American Optometric Association urges the schools and colleges of optometry to include education on issues relating to child abuse as part of their professional and continuing education curricula; and be it further

RESOLVED, that the American Optometric Association urges other providers of optometric continuing education programs to include education on issues relating to child abuse; and be it further

RESOLVED, that it is the responsibility of doctors of optometry, when they recognize evidence of child abuse, to refer and/or report such cases to appropriate authorities consistent with applicable federal, state, and local statutes.

1904 — EDUCATION IN ETHICS

(1 of 1994)   WHEREAS, a comprehensive understanding of ethics is essential for the humanitarian delivery of health care; and

WHEREAS, the practice of optometry must be firmly based on professional and moral ethics; and

WHEREAS, ethics education should be included within the formal optometric curricula of the schools and colleges of optometry; and

WHEREAS, optometric educators have begun to formulate a model curriculum on ethics; now therefore be it

RESOLVED, that the American Optometric Association endorses the study of ethics as an integral part of optometric education; and be it further

RESOLVED, that the American Optometric Association urges the schools and college of optometry, as well as its affiliate associations providing continuing education, to adopt structured curricula and programs in ethics.

1907 — AMERICANS WITH DISABILITIES ACT

(4 of 1994)   WHEREAS, the Americans with Disabilities Act provides a federal mandate which recognizes the need to accommodate persons with disabilities; and

WHEREAS, Doctors of Optometry must continue to be sensitive to and accessible for persons with disabilities; now therefore be it

RESOLVED, that the American Optometric Association urges schools and colleges of optometry, as well as affiliates of the American Optometric Association, to provide educational programs relating to the Americans with Disabilities Act for both students and Doctors of Optometry; and be it further

RESOLVED, that the American Optometric Association urges Doctors of Optometry to continue providing appropriate access to optometric care for persons with disabilities, as mandated by the Americans with Disabilities Act.

1908 VISION EXAMINATION OF SCHOOL-AGE CHILDREN

(Combination in 1995 of 1035-9 of 1953. - Mod. 1985 - and 1846-3 of 1986.- Mod. 1990)

WHEREAS, literature indicates that the visual process plays a vital role in learning, and any reduction in the efficiency of the visual system may result in the inability of children to achieve their full potential; and

WHEREAS, studies indicate that many school children have undetected, educationally significant visual problems;and

WHEREAS, optometrists are cognizant of and active in the field of vision as it relates to school achievement, and more optometrists are becoming interested and engaging in the field; and

WHEREAS, it is the responsibility of the optometrist to assess the school-age child's visual readiness for learning and the maintenance of visual performance; now therefore be it

RESOLVED, that the optometric examination of the school-age child should include appropriate recommendations to optimize visual function for classroom performance; and be it further

RESOLVED, that it is the responsibility of the optometrist to examine the eyes, analyze the functioning of the visual system, to prescribe lenses, prisms and vision therapy when necessary, and to collaborate with members of other professions which are also qualified to contribute to the growth, development and achievement of children.

1913	ETHICS COMMITTEE
(3 of 1995)	WHEREAS, significant changes in technology and in the delivery of optometric care and services are placing ever increasing burdens on the ethical and professional delivery of optometric care and services; now therefore be it

RESOLVED, that the affiliated associations of the American Optometric Association be encouraged to make efforts to raise the level of consciousness about issues of ethical behavior; to identify and address ethical concerns that relate to clinical practice; and to identify and address ethical concerns that relate to organizations' behavior; and be it further

RESOLVED, that the affiliated associations of the American Optometric Association be encouraged, with advice and guidance from their legal counsel, to activate committees on ethics and values which would address concerns as they may arise related to issues of ethical behavior in accordance with applicable federal and state laws.

1914	RELEASE OF PATIENT RECORDS
(4 of 1995)	WHEREAS, it is the professional and ethical responsibility of doctors of optometry to transmit to other professional

practitioners information from patient records upon written authorization by the patient; and

WHEREAS, the purpose of the transmittal of patient information to other practitioners is to provide all appropriate information for the continuity of care of the patient; and

WHEREAS, the patient may request and authorize the transmittal of only portions of their record; and

WHEREAS, deletion of portions of a patient's record may lead to false assumptions by the receiving professional practitioner, which may result in the potential harm of the patient; now therefore be it

RESOLVED, that doctors of optometry transmit to other professional practitioners, upon written authorization by the patient, all appropriate information as designated from the patient's record; and be it further

RESOLVED, that doctors of optometry transmitting patient records to another professional practitioner inform the practitioner when portions of a patient's record are being omitted at the request and authorization of the patient.

1916 (1 of 1996)   ABUSE AGAINST INDIVIDUALS UNABLE TO PROTECT THEMSELVES

WHEREAS, the awareness of abuse against individuals unable to protect themselves has been elevated to a level where society has taken increased steps to curtail the exploitation of these persons; and

WHEREAS, the profession of optometry has an ethical and societal responsibility to be advocates for those suffering abuse; now therefore be it

RESOLVED, that the American Optometric Association

and affiliated state associations be encouraged to provide members with educational resources to aid in the recognition of abuse against individuals unable to protect themselves; and be it further

RESOLVED, that the American Optometric Association encourage the National Board of Examiners in Optometry to include questions on the subject of abuse against individuals unable to protect themselves as a portion of their examination, making future practitioners more aware of these problems; and be it further

RESOLVED, that individual doctors of optometry be encouraged to report cases of suspected abuse to the appropriate authorities in accordance with current laws; and be it further

RESOLVED, that the American Optometric Association encourage all affiliated state associations to adopt a similar resolution.

1917   PROTECTING CONFIDENTIALITY DURING
(2 of 1996)   ELECTRONIC TRANSMISSION OF PATIENT
INFORMATION

WHEREAS, it is the professional and ethical responsibility of doctors of optometry to provide to other professional practitioners information from patient records upon written authorization by the patient; and

WHEREAS, sharing of patient clinical information for educational or other purposes may improve optometric care; and

WHEREAS, providing this information may be accomplished by utilizing widely accessible electronic media, such as the Internet; now therefore be it

RESOLVED, that doctors of optometry should take every reasonable precaution to protect a patient's identity, thereby maintaining confidentiality, when transmitting clinical information by electronic media.

1920 (5 of 1996)	DOCTOR/PATIENT COMMUNICATIONS IN MANAGED HEALTH CARE PLANS

WHEREAS, there is concern that some managed care contract clauses may limit doctors' ability to communicate with patients; and

WHEREAS, it is the ethical duty of doctors of optometry, as a fundamental element of the doctor-patient relationship, to act as an advocate on behalf of the patient; and

WHEREAS, it is a doctor's obligation to discuss necessary and appropriate treatment alternatives and in good faith to fully inform the patient of all treatment options; and

WHEREAS, the failure to communicate specific information may limit the patient's access to timely, relevant and quality health care services; now therefore be it

RESOLVED, that the American Optometric Association strongly encourages the adoption of federal legislation prohibiting managed care organizations from using restrictive contract clauses that may serve to limit a doctor's ability to communicate openly and freely with patients about their care options; and be it further

RESOLVED, that the American Optometric Association strongly encourages the affiliated state associations to seek the adoption of similar state legislation.

1923 (3 of 1997)	EYE AND VISION CARE FOR EVERY CHILD

WHEREAS, it is recognized that good eye and visual health is essential for the optimal development of every child; and

WHEREAS, doctors of optometry are recognized as primary eye and vision health care professionals who help assure maximum eye and visual health of children; now therefore be it

RESOLVED, that the American Optometric Association encourages doctors of optometry, as a matter of professional responsibility, to garner appropriate private and public support to assure that every child receives eye and vision care services essential for his or her optimal development.

1924 (4 of 1997) MAINTAINING HIGH STANDARDS FOR EYE AND VISION CARE

WHEREAS, the first precept of the Code of Ethics of the American Optometric Association requires doctors of optometry "to keep the visual welfare of the patient uppermost at all times"; and

WHEREAS, current conditions in health care often place additional constraints on health care providers; now therefore be it

RESOLVED, that the American Optometric Association affirms that doctors of optometry, as a matter of ethical concern, should continue to maintain high standards of eye and vision care such as set forth in the Optometric Clinical Practice Guidelines of the American Optometric Association.

Contributors

Arthur H. Alexander, OD

Dr. Alexander is Director of Optometry Programs at the Veterans Affairs Medical Center in Philadelphia and also maintains a private practice in that city. Dr. Alexander has held faculty appointments at the Southern California College of Optometry, the Pennsylvania College of Optometry, and the Pennsylvania College of Osteopathic Medicine, and he served as an optometrist in the U.S. Navy during the 1970s. He has been a member of the Ethics and Values Committee of the American Optometric Association. He has also served as a member of the ethics committees of Parkview Hospital and the Veterans Administration Hospital in Philadelphia. Dr. Alexander received the OD degree from the University of California, Berkeley.

R. Norman Bailey, MA, OD, MBA, MPH, FAAO

Dr. Bailey is an Associate Professor and member of the Attending Faculty of the University Eye Institute of the University of Houston College of Optometry. In addition to his clinical teaching, he lectures to professional students on topics in public health, health care organization, professionalism, and ethics. Dr. Bailey was in private optometric practice in Charlotte, North Carolina for ten years prior to joining the faculty at the University of Houston. He is a member of the Ethics and Values Committee of the American Optometric Association, currently serving as the Chair. In addition to being a Fellow of the American Academy of Optometry, he is a Diplomate of the Academy's Public Health Section. Dr. Bailey received the OD degree from Indiana University. He completed a Post-Doctoral Optometric Fellowship at the Gesell Institute of Child Development in New Haven, Connecticut.

Thomas F. Dorrity, Jr., OD

Dr. Dorrity is in private practice in Belleville, New Jersey. He is the current president of the New Jersey Society of Optometric Physicians and served as a member of their Board of Directors between 1985 and 1993. Dr. Dorrity was a member of the Ethics and Values Committee of the American Optometric Association from 1994 through 1998. He is a member of the Essex County Optometric Association, serving as their president from 1989 through 1992. He has served as a member of the Board of Trustees of the Pennsylvania College of Optometry. Dr. Dorrity was selected as the New Jersey Optometrist of the Year in 1997. He received the OD degree from the Pennsylvania College of Optometry.

Kia B. Eldred, OD, FAAO

Dr. Eldred is an Assistant Visiting Professor at the University of Houston College of Optometry. She is a member of the Attending Faculty at the University Eye Institute's Non-Invasive Objective Visual Assessment Clinic for Multi-handicapped Patients and Vision Rehabilitation Services, and at the Institute for Rehabilitation. Dr. Eldred has been the Course-Master for the Vision Rehabilitation Course at the University of Houston for the past eight years. She has served as the Director of the Lighthouse of Houston Low Vision Clinic and as Director of External Education at the University of Houston College of Optometry. In addition to being a Fellow of the American Academy of Optometry, she is a Diplomate of the Academy's Low Vision Section. Dr. Eldred received the OD degree from the University of Houston.

N. Scott Gorman, OD, MS, FAAO

Dr. Gorman is a Professor at the Nova Southeastern University College of Optometry. Prior to joining the faculty, Dr. Gorman was in private optometric practice for thirteen years, limiting his practice to nursing home residents. He served on the professional staffs of twenty skilled nursing facilities in the south Florida area. He is a member of the Miami Area Geriatric Education Center's Executive Committee, and Chair of the Nursing Home and Geriatric Practice Committees of the Florida and American Optometric Associations. In addition to being a Fellow of the American Academy of Optometry, he is a Diplomate and the Chair of the Academy's Optometric Education Section. Dr. Gorman received the OD degree from the Southern College of Optometry.

Elizabeth Heitman, PhD

Dr. Heitman is Associate Professor of Ethics in Health Care at the University of Texas-Houston School of Public Health. She teaches ethics across the UT-Health Science Center, including courses in theoretical and clinical medical ethics, ethics in the biomedical sciences, and public health ethics, and serves on the institutional ethics committees of a number of Houston-area hospitals. Dr. Heitman regularly participates as a visiting lecturer in the course "Community Health Optometry" at the University of Houston College of Optometry, and has been a consultant to the AOA's Ethics and Values Committee since 1994. Between 1989 and 1994 she served as the Assistant Editor of the International Journal of Technology Assessment in Health Care, and from 1994 through 1999 served as the Associate Editor. Dr. Heitman received the PhD degree from the Department of Religious Studies at Rice University, with specialization in medical ethics and medical anthropology.

Elizabeth Hoppe, OD, MPH, DrPH, FAAO

Dr. Hoppe is an Associate Professor at the Southern California College of Optometry where she teaches in the low vision and public health curricula. She is the Director of Outcomes Research at SCCO. Dr. Hoppe also serves as the Coordinator for the Foothill Center for the Partially Sighted. She is a member of the Information and Data Committee of the AOA, and Chair-Elect of the Vision Care Section Council of the American Public Health Association. In addition to being a Fellow of the American Academy of Optometry, she is a Diplomate of the Academy's Public Health Section. Dr. Hoppe received the OD degree from Ferris State University and the DrPH degree from the University of Michigan.

Dawn C. Kaufman, OD

Dr. Kaufman is in private optometric practice in Freeman, South Dakota with her husband, LeRoy Kaufman, OD. She has a special interest in the areas of optometric practice serving the visual needs of children and the care of contact lens patients. She has served as President of the South Dakota Optometric Society and of the North Central States Optometric Council. She has been a Trustee of the American Optometric Association, serving as the Secretary-Treasurer of the AOA from 1994-1995. She received the Indiana University Foley House Award in 1996. Dr. Kaufman received the OD degree from Indiana University.

LeRoy Kaufman, OD

Dr. Kaufman is in private optometric practice in Freeman, South Dakota with his wife, Dawn Kaufman, OD. He has served as President of the South Dakota Optometric Society. Dr. Kaufman has been a member of the South Dakota State Board of Examiners. He has been a member of the AOA Statutory Definition Committee and served on the AOA Council on Optometric Education. Dr. Kaufman was named the South Dakota Optometrist of the Year in 1991 and received the South Dakota Distinguished Service award in 1996. He was a member of the South Dakota Legislature from 1972 – 1976. Dr. Kaufman received the OD degree from Indiana University.

Brian S. Klinger, OD, FAAO

Dr. Klinger is in private optometric practice in Portsmouth, New Hampshire. He has served as President of the New Hampshire Optometric Association, President of the New England Council of Optometrists, and as Trustee and Secretary-Treasurer of the American Optometric Association. He has been a member of numerous committees, including the Ethics and Values Committee of the AOA. Dr. Klinger currently serves as President and member of the Board of Directors of the International Library, Archives and Museum of Optometry in St. Louis. He is a Fellow of the American Academy of Optometry. Dr. Klinger received the OD degree from the Illinois College of Optometry.

Michael Larkin, OD, FAAO

Dr. Larkin is in private practice in Los Alamitos, California. He is an Assistant Professor at the Southern California College of Optometry. Dr. Larkin is Past-Chair of the AOA's Eye Care Benefits Center and currently the Center's Chair of the Subcommittee on Coding. He serves on the AMA's Health Care Professions Advisory Panel for CPT and is a member of the AMA CPT-5 Workgroup. Dr. Larkin served with Dr. William Hsiao on his Technical Consulting Group for the Harvard School of Public Health on the issue of E/M coding. He is the inventor of the pharmaceutical combination known as Paremyd. He is a Fellow of the American Academy of Optometry. Dr. Larkin received the OD degree from the Southern California College of Optometry.

Edwin C. Marshall, OD, MS, MPH, FAAO

Dr. Marshall is a Professor of Optometry and the Associate Dean for Academic Affairs at the Indiana University School of Optometry. In addition to being very active in a number of public health activities, he serves on the boards of directors of the Indiana Optometric Association and the Indiana Public Health Association. He is a Past Chair of the Vision Care Section Council of the American Public Health Association. Dr. Marshall has been a recipient of the Distinguished Service to Optometry Award of the Indiana Optometric Association and has received special recognition from the Indiana Public Health Association. In addition to being a Fellow of the American Academy of Optometry, he is a Diplomate of the Academy's Public Health Section. Dr. Marshall received the OD degree from Indiana University.

David T. Ozar, PhD

Dr. Ozar is Professor and Co-Director of Graduate Studies in Health Care Ethics in the Department of Philosophy at Loyola University of Chicago, and Director of Loyola's Center for Ethics. He is also Adjunct Professor of Medical Humanities in Loyola's Stritch School of Medicine. He has taught in many of the professional school programs at Loyola since 1972. In addition, Dr. Ozar is an associate member of the professional staff, associate director of the medical ethics program, member of the institutional ethics committee, and consulting ethicist at Evanston Hospital in Evanston, Illinois. He has served as a consultant to professional committees, organizations, and schools, including the Ethics and Values Committee of the AOA and the American Dental Association. Dr. Ozar received the PhD degree in philosophy from Yale University.

Mark Swanson, OD, FAAO

Dr. Swanson is an Associate Professor of Optometry at the University of Alabama at Birmingham School of Optometry. He has appointments as a Scientist in the University of Alabama's Center for Aging, Center for Health Promotion, and Vision Science Research Center. His current area of research interest is mobility and falls in the elderly. His research is funded through the U.S. Centers for Disease Control and Prevention. He currently serves on the AOA Hospital, Nursing Home, and Geriatric Committee. Dr. Swanson is a Fellow of the American Academy of Optometry. Dr. Swanson received the OD degree from the University of Alabama at Birmingham.

Satya B. Verma, OD, FAAO

Dr. Verma is Director of Resident Eye Care at the Pennsylvania College of Optometry. He is a member and Past Chair of the Professional Relations Committee of the American Optometric Association. He chaired the Vision Care Section of the American Public Health Association in 1999. Dr. Verma has served as President of the Pennsylvania Optometric Association and is currently serving on Association committees. He is a member of the Board of the National Council on Aging. Dr. Verma was the 1998 American Optometric Association's Optometrist of the Year. He received the same award from his local and state optometric associations in previous years. He has been presented the Distinguished Service Award by Prevent Blindness, America. In addition to being a Fellow of the American Academy of Optometry, he is a Diplomate of the Academy's Public Health Section. Dr. Verma received the OD degree from the Pennsylvania College of Optometry and the D.R.Opt. from the School of Optometry, Gandhi Eye Hospital, Aligarh, India.

Siu G. Wong, OD, MPH, FAAO

Dr. Wong is the Managed Care Specialist, USPHS-Indian Health Service (IHS) Albuquerque Area and Director, Division of Eye Care, IHS Albuquerque Area. Prior to joining the IHS, she taught for five years at the University of Houston College of Optometry. In addition, Dr Wong has been appointed a member and/or chair of various committees of the American Optometric Association, the American Academy of Optometry, and the American Public Health Association. She has received numerous awards and commendations from the U.S. Public Health Service. She was selected the New Mexico Woman Optometrist in 1984. Dr. Wong is a Fellow of the American Academy of Optometry. Dr. Wong received the OD degree from the University of California, Berkeley.